the

Experts' Acclaim for *Moving Your Aging Parents*

"*Moving Your Aging Parents* is a creative and inspiring godsend for helping Mom and Dad transition to the next phase of life. Nancy shows us how to heal ourselves, talk to each other, make plans, organize, pack, move, and create a new home and life to thrive—not merely survive. Valuable for caregivers, healthcare professionals, and seniors interested in aging with independence, dignity and grace."   —Jacqueline Marcell,
                 author *Elder Rage*, host *Coping With Caregiving* radio show

"Nancy Wesson has tackled successfully one of the most difficult areas of caring for aging parents: helping them retain a sense of their own space and their own place. Her practical, do-able approach will help baby boomers avoid mistakes and make their parents feel at home wherever they may be. As a veteran of 12 years of parent care, I recommend this book highly."   —Jim Comer,
            author *When Roles Reverse: A Guide to Parenting Your Parents*

"*Moving Your Aging Parents* is an excellent guidebook for anyone who is engaged in the process of orchestrating the downsizing and relocation of another human being, whether a parent (the actual subject of this book), another loved one, or even themselves. The author has drawn widely from respected experts in a diverse field of disciplines, and has truly created a reference book for managing environment to create a special place of retreat. The special needs of the aging or disabled are thoughtfully considered, with practical solutions for overcoming barriers related to diminished hearing, vision, dexterity, strength, ambulation ability, as well as mental capacity and memory.

"As a thirty-five year plus veteran of health care practice as a Registered Nurse, specializing in the care of the elderly, I offer my heart-felt endorsement of this excellent book. It offers concrete plans to follow and emphasizes the emotional and spiritual counterparts that transform seemingly difficult chores into acts of mutual joy, growth, and love."
                                         —Mary Durfor, *Rebecca's Reads*

"As founder of an integrative health care practice, I specialize in the care of the elderly from a mind, body, spirit perspective. Life transitions management is a large part of this work... Nancy's approach is both genuine and practical, offering a valuable tool for this very important and often neglected phase of life."   —Chris Holland, PhD, FNP, RN
Contemporary Health Care, Austin, Texas

"...a thoughtful and intelligent guide helpful not only to family members, but anyone involved with their situation. The information in *Moving Your Aging Parents* is relevant for every relocation regardless of the age or circumstances of the client. "
—Sally B. Yaryan, Director, Professional Development & Education,
Austin Board of REALTORS®

"...a poignant, sensitive account...a guidebook not only to the compassionate treatment of elders but also for seniors themselves as they face making choices on their own"   —Diana M. DeLuca, Ph.D.,
author, *Seniors Dealing with Life*, http://coololdtech.blogspot.com

"This is a must-read book for anyone helping their aging parents. Nancy Wesson has taken the precepts of Feng Shui, adapted them in wonderful and practical ways and applied them with such deep compassion. Readers will find so many useful tips and strategies and will also learn much more about themselves in the process."
—Lillian Garnier Bridges, President, Lotus Institute, Inc.
author *Face Reading in Chinese Medicine*

"Having just spent a week with my 83 year-old mother, I realized that there were many changes in her life that I was not aware of. Ms. Wesson's book gave me plenty of ideas of how to approach a move with my mother. Stubborn as my mom is I was able to handle this with few disagreements. As an advocate for Concerned Citizens to Protect the Elderly for many years, this is a book I recommended to the committee to get plenty of help for children of the elderly. As a college instructor for nurses, this is a book I put on recommended reading. Thank you Ms. Wesson."
—Reviewed by Carol Hoyer, Ph.D. Family Psychology

MOVING YOUR AGING PARENTS

Fulfilling Their Needs and Yours
Before, During and After the Move

Nancy Daniel Wesson

For reprinted text permission statements, please see page iv.

Library of Congress Cataloging-in-Publication Data

Wesson, Nancy Daniel, 1947-
 Moving your aging parents : fulfilling their needs and yours before, during, and after the move / Nancy Daniel Wesson.
   p. cm.
 Includes bibliographical references and index.
 ISBN-13: 978-1-932690-54-5 (trade paper : alk. paper)
 ISBN-10: 1-932690-54-9 (trade paper : alk. paper)
 1. Aging parents--Care. 2. Adult children of aging parents--Family relationships.
3. Aging parents--Family relationships. I. Title.
 HQ1063.6.W47 2008
 306.88--dc22

2008003375

Also available in fine hardcover editions:
ISBN-13: 978-1-61599-013-9 (hardcover : alk. paper)
ISBN-10: 1-61599-013-5 (hardcover : alk. paper)

Distributed by:
Quality Books, Ingram Book Group, New Leaf Distributing

Published by:
Loving Healing Press
5145 Pontiac Trail
Ann Arbor, MI 48105
USA

http://www.LovingHealing.com or
email info@LovingHealing.com
Tollfree 888-761-6268
Fax 734-663-6861

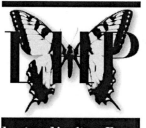

Dedication

To my mother, Lee Daniel—
for all the obvious reasons,
and even more that aren't

Table of Contents

Diagrams

Permissions

We gratefully acknowledge receiving permission from the following individuals and groups for quotations provided in this text. In alphabetical order:

Richard A. Amen, M.D. from *Change your brain, change your life* (courtesy of Random House).

Brian Green from *The Elegant Universe* (courtesy of W.W. Norton & Co.)

"Symphony" by Daniel H. Pink, from *A Whole New Mind* by Daniel Pink, copyright © 2005 by Daniel H. Pink. Used by permission of Riverhead Books, an imprint of Penguin Group (USA) Inc.

"Watch Lights" from Lillian Phillips, LCSW, Innovative Senior Care/ Brookdale Senior Living and Terry Rauschuber, LCSW, Heritage Program for Senior Adults.

Thomas-Kilman Conflict Mode Instrument (courtesy of CPP, Inc., see add'l. note on p. 65)

David Wolfe from *Ageless Marketing* blog.

From *Getting To Yes, 2/e* by Roger Fisher, William Ury, and Bruce Patton. Copyright © 1981, 1991 by Roger Fisher and William Ury. Reprinted by permission of Houghton Mifflin Harcourt Publishing Company. All rights reserved.

Foreword

This book is a treasure trove of practical tools, valuable insights and heartfelt hope. Nancy shares her eldercare experience (which most of us will have with our own aging parents) through rich and honest stories and practical, compassionate guidance centered around moving her own mother. Through creative techniques developed over decades of working with clients and students, she not only shows us how to help our parents' transition to their new life, but offers a sensitive guide for creating a whole new way for living it.

Early on, Nancy makes the statement that "After physical needs are met, this endeavor [moving our parents] has far more to do with the spirit than at any other time of life." Far from offering platitudes, Nancy offers a valuable, heretofore unavailable blend of practicality and inspiration. Her real-life stories are profoundly moving, but she doesn't take the easy road and stop there. She offers us the real tools—all practical, some original, some taken from other research and disciplines and exquisitely adapted to this phase of life. Some are geared to getting our parents on board and engaged in the possibilities; others act as a lifeline to pull us, their children and helpers, out of the quicksand of competing responsibilities and make it possible to help with grace and wisdom.

At the core of such transitions are deeply conflicting feelings and the need to communicate from the heart. But schedules, fears, old wounds, personal needs, grief, fear and egos act as obstacles to our providing the comfort and support we intend. Nancy offers very specific techniques and skills to guide us through not only the difficult conversations with our parents, but our own internal dialogues as well. She offers deep insight into the divergent histories that have created the often-conflicting mindsets and values that make even talking about this move so heart-wrenching. Nancy's understanding of these issues and the guidance she provides offer us a way to be gentle with our parents and still move forward with the task at hand. Her shared experiences with her mother and her clients are proof that it is possible to transform this event. Instead of it being on-the-job-training which we must endure and survive, it really can be a positive, life-healing experience—ushering us into an increasingly rich and fulfilling adult relationship with our parents.

The processes presented in this book apply even if we are not physically relocating our parents. They are just as appropriate when applied to a new stage of life in their own homes. Her book offers a great many things we can do to help them age-in-place and remain at home longer—maintaining their dignity and independence as long as possible and on their terms. In the chapter on Special Needs, Nancy identifies behavioral characteristics to help with early identification of some of the maladies that complicate later life and have been at the root of premature nursing home placements. There are many simple environmental adjustments that can make life easier and safer for those living with hearing loss, arthritis, dementia, Parkinson's or low-vision. In addition to nurturing autonomy and personal dignity, they might well defer a move into more restrictive accommodations.

One of the comments I hear repeatedly in working in the realm of eldercare is that "Mom and Dad are just not adjusting well to the move." Most books stop with "moving in." This book goes far beyond and uses diagrams and stories to show us how to set-up the new residence and help them feel "at home." Her ideas about re-claiming daily rituals to help them bond with their new lives are compelling. And the tips on where to go and who to contact to help our folks build new connections and friendships are true lifesavers.

Nancy is a believer that quality of life and quality of environment are inseparable and she shows us with amazing clarity how thought, emotions and environment combine to help people create emotionally rich and sustaining lives regardless of circumstances or age. She shows us how to work with what we have, and turn the-hand-we-have-been-dealt into one that serves us and those we love throughout and long after the physical transition.

Nancy has a unique ability to merge a wide range of seemingly divergent topics and skills into a whole that not only makes sense, but is inspirational. With compassion, humor and insight she tackles conflict resolution, spirituality, organization, interior design, space-planning (Feng Shui) and special needs—and presents the whole lot in an orderly, logical manner. In doing so she expertly guides us around every eldercare obstacle, while teaching us how to effectively communicate and negotiate with loved ones born of a different era. Ultimately she leads the reader through a process of discovery that can be life-changing. By the end of the book we realize this book goes far beyond just the task or relocating: it offers a blueprint for living a purpose driven life.

Jacqueline Marcell,
Author of *Elder Rage!: How to Survive Caring for Aging Parents*
host of the *Coping With Caregiving* radio show

Acknowledgements

The working title for this book was My Mother's Chair, but that title died on the Google vine, because no one would know how to search for the book. Nevertheless, it does point the way to the first and most important "thank you" for this entire project. My mother modestly played the central character of this book and "her chair," the supporting role. Because of the several moves we have accomplished together, each new event became a chapter, each failed communication became a subheading, and each effort to find a new pathway around a problem found its way into an exercise at the end of a chapter.

Without a doubt, however, the greatest gift was the sweet relationship that evolved during this deeply personal process. As is true for many mothers and daughters, my mother and I certainly have had our issues and unresolved conflicts masterfully buried under years of avoidance, work-arounds, moves, births, deaths, divorces and ultimately my becoming an adult with children of my own. Truly, this process of ushering her into her elder-phase of life gave birth to a relationship filled with greater understanding of the other, mutual compassion, deep insights into what made us both tic and ultimately healing of the old wounds and misunderstandings. No, we were not free of conflict. We just handled it differently and acknowledged each other in the process. She learned how to apologize, I learned how "not to confront." We laughed together and we cried, but mostly we loved. This healing spread into every other aspect of our lives. She, for perhaps the first time in her life, was able to taste the sweetness life has to offer. It is never too late.

To Evie, my sister, thanks for hours of conversation unraveling our common history. As you have lovingly said, "I laugh because you are my sister, and there's nothing you can do about it!"

Additional help flowed in from so many different and sometimes, unlikely, sources. Dick, my Dad, has been gone many years now, but seemed always present. So often I could hear his chuckle or see the shrug of his shoulders when things got interesting. Pat Barnes, my friend and gifted artist, painstakingly read the first draft in its entirety and offered comments in that tactful southern way that never bruised or offended, yet always improved the final product. Moreover, her encouragement kept the book going when life derailed it.

Catherine Hastings' contributions have been incalculable. After reading the first five chapters of the book Cathy offered to do the cover and the illustrations. She is a genius at doing things I consider impossible and has an uncanny knack for being able to capture the essence of person's thoughts and emotions and put them into a logo, web-site, illustration or piece of art. She designed the cover and the illustrations on the website with no guidance from me and I believe the results speak for themselves.

Thanks to Irene Watson for believing in the book and for making the connection to Victor Volkman, my publisher. For a first time author, this was a stunning synchronicity. Thank you, Victor. To Bob Rich, my Aussie editor—in spite my complaints about formatting changes—thanks for teaching me more than I really wanted to know about the use of "find and replace." Your editing was priceless, but your sidebar commentary about how you liked this phrase or that and your philosophical musings made the process a partnership. If this book reads with an Aussie accent, you can thank Bob.

My deepest love and appreciation go to my two sons, Travis and Brett, both great adventuresome young men finding their own bright paths. Your abiding faith, good humor and willingness to be guinea pigs as I arranged and re-arranged your rooms, lectured you on the power of thought to guide life and required you to mediate your own brotherly disputes ultimately transformed all our lives. You are the shining lights of my life.

Love to you all!

Introduction

The idea for this book came to me while driving back from a visit with my 85-year-old mother. This was the second time I'd helped her recover her home after it had been broken into and robbed by vandals while she was traveling. This time, they simply removed the back sliding-glass door (locks intact), walked in and rummaged through her belongings until they found anything they could use or fence. As a Feng Shui consultant and a professional organizer, I've gentled many clients through the process of organizing greater chaos than this. But working with my own mother was light years removed from the less intimate process of helping hundreds of clients with whom I have no deep emotional bonds, complicated history or family responsibility.

This time it was Mom and she was angry, confused, adrift and vulnerable. While organizing for another person is always an intimate and surprisingly emotional process because of the personal nature of the information shared, this same process with my mother tipped the scales. It was to be a precursor of things to come—moving her into a *retirement complex* closer to me. We both know it is probably the last place she will call "home." It came at a time when I had just made my own move back to my Texas roots, down-sizing and settling in for my own "next stage." Unlike my work with clients, this sequence of events unleashed long dormant emotions and a few new ones I hadn't even suspected were germinating.

My mother's life and mine are hinged together at the core, and every decision we make together is a negotiation; every decision I make alone is loaded with an assumption that I know what is best for her and the realization that—if I am wrong—there might be hell to pay later for one of us. I want to "do right" by my mother, but I am wearing many clashing hats: her little girl, a seasoned professional who does this for a living and the new and odd role as parent of my parent. As we desperately tried to find the documents the insurance company demanded before it would support her claim, part of my brain fast forwarded to the future when I may be called upon to find financial documents, medical records, title to the house, etc. Although documents were in a worse than normal state of chaos, it became clear that she had never had a coherent system and important papers had been stashed in little nests all over the house. She had also secreted-away the silverware and other valuables in hiding places in the back of kitchen cabinets and God knows where else. The thieves obviously knew this tendency of older folks to hide things, because they even dismantled parts of the attic looking for treasures.

Why didn't I know this about her?

Her house had become a shrine to all the memories of a life gone by: one where picking cotton and selling tomatoes earned her college tuition at LSU where she met and married my dad—a handsome, free spirit. I found his picture again and again—this time standing in front of a B-52 bomber looking like Clark Gable in fatigues. After thirty-plus years of marriage and my father's death, there were more recent pictures of her in a newly crafted solo existence. Some were pictures of her birding in Costa Rica. Others were from her period of volunteering in remote sections of Big Bend, the source of the her stories of picking up the pieces after drug-deals-gone-wrong resulted in bodies—dead and alive—deposited at her doorstep. How do you go from such an independent and adventurous life to being the victim of break-ins and your daughter moving you into safer terrain?

You just age, that's how.

As baby boomers, we ourselves are aging. There—I've said it and it's still ringing in my ears. Not only are we moving our parents into the next stage, WE are trying to find our way through a process for which the paradigm is just now being created. We are pioneers in constructing a new approach to aging that is defined by active lifestyles and more open relationships with our children, coupled with a shifting financial terrain and at-risk social security. While *active-lifestyle* retirement communities are one of the fastest growing businesses in the U.S., there remains a scarcity of tools at our fingertips. This book is offered both as a shared experience and a guide to navigating this new terrain.

At the heart of the journey is creating a sense of place, whether it is for our parents or ourselves. This is soul work. It transcends the process of finding health care, safety and "good help," all of which keep us alive, but not thriving. That's the job of *environments* that feed the emotions and *connections* that keep the spirit alive and well nourished. All are essential to life. To ignore the latter and keep one alive in the absence of emotionally engaging surroundings is to starve the spirit, the essence of life and well-being. Starving the spirit results in anger, depression, a feeling of helplessness and ultimately the loss of the will to live. It sucks the lifeblood and leaves those who have given their lives over to doctors' appointments, walkers and nursing care lost in a land of foreigners, people who frequently don't listen, and when they do, they seldom hear. The body is safe, but the soul hungers. (If you are uncertain about your parent's need for additional help or a change in living circumstances, the list provided in the Appendix should provide you with some cues.)

As we grew up, my mother shared with us her favorite poem. In trying to recall the circumstances of its being mentioned, I remember that we always had flowers around the house: gladiolas, pansies, zinnias, gardenias, bottlebrush and camellias. At some point, as I was leaving to set up my own home, she reminded me to always have flowers, even if I had to take money away from something else. Here is the poem:

> If of thy mortal goods thou art bereft,
> And from thy slender store two loaves
> alone to thee are left,
> Sell one, and with the dole
> Buy hyacinths to feed thy soul.
> > Moslih Eddin Saadi, *Gulistan*
> > *(Garden of Roses)*

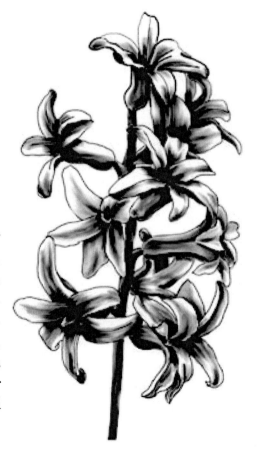

Helping an elderly parent downsize and go through a process that we, ourselves, are loath to do is *not the same* as guiding someone who is upwardly mobile and enjoying the climb. The realities of divesting and de-cluttering, both actions you may have initiated in the past, are different. The process bears some similarities in mechanics, but not in emotions. Managing these emotions, supporting the day-to-day practicalities with soul and beauty, and enriching your relationship with your self and your loved ones are the goals of this book.

I have seen the devastating consequences of well-meaning friends and children going through Mom's and Dad's belongings without realizing the fragile nature of what they were doing. Trust is destroyed, feelings hurt, relationships damaged at the very time in life we have the least opportunity to repair them and our hearts ache to give our parents what they need.

These are crucial times for us all. We can choose whether we merely survive, or whether we thrive by moving forward with grace, insight and humor. The tools and insights offered in this book will guide you through the process of creating a life for yourself or your parent that is characterized by insight in the face of challenge, grace in the process of aging, empathy in the midst of conflict, and beauty in the presence of functionality.

1

My Mother's Chair

Rain is slamming against the windshield and I can't see the edge of I-10 that runs through the swamp west of Lake Charles. I'm only an hour out so it seems a waste to find a hotel. I can't even call mom to let her know I'll be late because I can't risk the distraction. It's all I can do to keep my little Subaru WRX on the road; even the all-wheel drive is being challenged by the wall of water shoving me sideways—delivered by an eighteen-wheeler that just barreled by. There is a sense of urgency about this trip as mom has finally made the decision to consider a move nearer to me. My sister and I have decided to alternate trips to her home to start the inevitable process of clearing things out in an effort to be ready to move to a smaller place. This is the first foray into that unknown territory.

Her agreement to move to a retirement complex near me (sometime in the next six months or so are her terms) has been nothing if not miraculous, but as luck would have it, her unit has become available early—four months early actually. The decision to take the unit had to be made now or wait another year, so we are beginning the process and my trip over to her represents the first step into the reality that she can a no longer manage on her own. How has it come to this so quickly? It seems that only last year she was talking about another rigorous trip to Costa Rica.

I am struggling to stay on the road while I wonder what stormy weather lies ahead in terms of this new stage. Further, I don't have time for this week away from a consulting business that depends on my personal presence to keep me funded. I've just relocated back to Austin after the realization that the move to West Virginia, while it was right at the time, is not right five years later. I've moved back to my "tribe" and I am just getting my business ramped up.

Realities of Aging

A year earlier, I had made this trip to help mom recover from *another* break-in, the first one having occurred nine years ago in the Baton Rouge home, where I grew up. It was the event that prompted the move to a *safer* neighborhood, closer to family, in Lake Charles.

On one level, I am superbly suited to help her. Helping people organize, move, create comfortable spaces for themselves and make life changes is my professional life. I love doing it and I'm good at it. But doing it for Mom was loaded with all manner of emotional baggage. I remembered some of it from the previous move, but that was just to a new city near friends (and excellent birding) and a more manageable house. She was in her mid seventies then, the landscape was different and she was more resilient. This time, she was unhinged and feeling victimized on many levels. The balance between intimacy and detachment possible with clients totally disintegrated in the presence of her despair. If I allowed myself to get enmeshed in the grief, it derailed the progress we needed to make. If I detached, it ignored her need for connection and my ability to listen with my heart. The same compassion, patience, tact and humor spontaneously present with others, became intermingled with anger, fear, frustration, old roles, expectations and a sense of impending doom that comes from knowing that every decision made would impact our relationship, as well as her health and independence. Yes, her situation could have been far worse: things could have been torn up beyond any reasonable repair; she could have been home during the attack. We both took some consolation in the fact that most of the items taken could be replaced, but that doesn't begin to cover the sense of being victimized or the loss of irreplaceable, sentimental items. The realization that there would be less time in the future to make new memories and that we were in a time warp propelling us both forward into the realities of aging—hers and mine—was profoundly sobering, and foreshadowed things to come.

The Clock is Ticking

During this process, it occurred to me that while the circumstances of my helping her were unique, the skills and processes are similar any time we help a parent, loved one or ourselves move through the pivotal drama of relocating in the later stages of life. The feelings of compassion and the emotional, psychological and spiritual tools needed to re-create a supportive space are essential to any process where there are life-altering transitions. As a nation of baby boomers, many of us have already navigated the "empty-nest" syndrome, are considering more efficient (cost and time) life styles, or facing the challenge of helping our parents relocate into smaller, more manageable surroundings and sometimes nursing homes. Moving is a tricky process regardless, but some of us are in the unenviable position of moving ourselves AND moving our parents. Moving our parents requires a unique toolset because we are straddling a paradigm chasm that spans everything from a shift in consciousness to knowing how to navigate cyberspace. We are speaking different languages and sometimes we need a translator. While our parents are dealing with the loss of options and autonomy, we are hell-bent to keep ours. And moving our parents scares the daylights out of us because the clock is ticking...

Making Sense of It All

Although we may not be dealing with theft in the literal sense, emotions and feelings of loss—whether it's letting go of items held onto for a lifetime or shifts in family dynamics—run rampant during this stage. The parent can suffer other losses, including the erosion of autonomy, which can result from diminished physical or mental capacity, the feelings of violation that come from having to leave one's home for a facility, or the need to downsize or relocate for any number of reasons.

The personal nature of this thrust me into a different framework of thinking and feeling my way through the process, using every tool at my disposal. Since the first vandalism, we have traveled through the second break-in and two relocations to different states and radically different "states-of-mind." Most recently, she has moved from a larger home in a city she's come to know, to the retirement complex, where everything is new, including the concept of renting, not having her garden, or even knowing how to get to the nearest K-Mart.

My mother is financially stable but not wealthy, and had little of value. During the break-in they took televisions, radios, yard tools and a handful of silver jewelry with more sentimental than monetary value. Evidently they knew that many elderly people hide their valuables in unlikely places like the pantry, the attic, in books, etc., and ransacked her closets, drawers—even the air conditioner housing in the attic—to see where she might be hiding the "good stuff." In the process, they also upended boxes and cabinets with legal documents, medical history, bill payments, etc. It's the kind of thing you don't think too much about, until you're faced with the task of making sense of it all—and locating the documents required by the insurance company to file a claim! The same is true when families come in after a health crisis or any number of events embedded in the tapestry of elder-life.

The emotional and physical processes involved with elder-moves are distinctly different from working with other stages of life and with the "thirty-something" population still raising their families, still accumulating, still actively building their resources and still essentially independent. Personal relocations after age 60, and especially those of geriatric parents, require a sensitivity and awareness to a uniquely amassing and shifting set of needs and concerns related to aging, health, cognition, mobility, independence and place in community. *After physical needs are met, this endeavor has far more to do with the spirit than at any other time of life.*

What Matters Most

The process of helping my mother regain control of her home and her life required asking the question, "what matters most," over and over again in a million different ways.

- What brings joy to everyday living?

- What is working—what is not?

- What level of access is needed for medications, phone numbers, medical records, etc.?

- What losses or perceived losses is she experiencing?

- What does she need more of? Less of?

- How do we address mobility issues?

- How are her senses functioning and what is needed to accommodate changes in acuity?

- How can I nourish the quality of life on a moment-to-moment basis and make access to those vital activities, items and places easy for her?

- What will she need in order to integrate into and build a new community—one that encourages staying connected, builds new friendships and sustains a *joie-de-vivre?*

Normal Redefined

We had to make many choices, and each required attention to how it felt. It seemed endless. In the process, I began to learn and value things about my mother that I'd never really thought about before. I began to know her in a different way, and therefore, began to be able to honor her in the ways I might have missed without the intimacy that results from dealing with real need or tragedy. As the process continued, I did better at this some days than on others. Honoring her became more subtle and encapsulated in the way questions were asked or answered, in dealing with her responses or lack of the same, and in replacing judgment or personal agendas with patience, gentleness, clarity and acceptance, and the ability to know when to "shut up and listen." It's actually easier to do this when one is in the midst of crisis, because anyone can be focused and compassionate in spurts. Maintaining it over the long haul is the tricky part. As we become re-entrenched in the details of our daily lives, it's natural to slip back into old patterns—fooling ourselves into thinking that once the move is over, things will normalize. And they do to a degree, but "normal" also becomes redefined. Settling into a new place, making friends, learning the ways around a new town takes a while—a least a year. That year was but a hiccup in time in our thirties and forties. By the time you're in your eighties, a year becomes disproportionately huge when viewed in the context of the lifetime remaining!

Command Central

In the process of putting things back in order after the break-in or creating order where none had been in the first place, it became apparent that her entire life revolved around a central element: *her chair.* No, she is not confined to that chair, nor is it a wheelchair. It is, however command central. Let me explain… It was banked on both sides by library bookracks on wheels so they could be pulled closer with ease—each holding three to four shelves of reference books for crossword puzzles. Add to that, glasses, writing materials, telephone, Kleenex, speakerphone (easier with her hearing aid), phone books, remotes and several sets of binoculars. Did I mention she's a birdwatcher? This chair and its strategic placement with easy access to her back door constituted the single most important aspect of her 1500 square foot home. It overlooked six bird feeders, the deck strewn with only the finest black-oil sunflower seeds, numerous watering stations, and hoses (and water-cannons to squirt birdseed-eating squirrels). This chair retained its importance in her new, abbreviated space, and its strategic placement remained paramount.

A Life Worth Living

The chair and its accoutrements represent a life worth living. It's not JUST a chair. As a former reference librarian and the director of a metropolitan library's children's room, she is both driven and sustained by her knowledge of thousands of bits of information. She breezes through the New York Times crossword puzzles and acrostics like some people devour potato chips. This particular hobby:

- Provides the mental exercise to keep her brain sharper than most 30-year-olds';

- Keeps her connected with current events;

- Wards off Alzheimer's; and

- Makes her one of the best conversationalists I've ever met.

An avid ornithologist, she's been studying and trekking off to spy on her feathered friends since I was in the sixth grade. Birds and puzzles are not just her FUN. They add years to her life, as well as enhance her ability to retain an independent life style and care for herself. How so?

- Bending and stooping to feed and water her birds and hiking to watch them gave the physical movement crucial to simultaneously oxygenate the brain, and to keep the cerebellum (containing 90% of the brains neural network) healthy;

- Staying active kept her body flexible and moving, reducing the likelihood of incapacitating injury;

- To this day, constant learning has kept her engaged with life and ideas; and

- Birding trips (like bridge, hunting, and sporting events) created a context for social outings.

These points are emphasized to remind us that every decision, whether made consciously or through default (not acting), has a consequence. While moving her to a less demanding lifestyle was necessary in one context, it has also removed the very things that caused her to be active. Ignoring the significance of the chair could have dire consequences in that its existence, ergonomics, and placement have impacted her ability to maintain an activity that is life sustaining.

What Makes the Heart Sing?

This single piece of furniture, seemingly ordinary to the untrained eye, became a metaphor symbolizing the importance of finding out what makes the heart sing for yourself or your parent and bringing it to life, so that the quality of life transcends the ordinary. Finding that "something" for yourself or your parent makes the difference between simply surviving and thriving. It goes beyond function and aesthetics as well as our own concepts of what is of value. It begs time, interest, insight, active listening, and patience.

So let's talk more about this chair, because the care taken in actually *choosing* it is demonstrative of the layers of awareness and attention brought to the process of consciously selecting what travels with us on the journey to the next place and configuring the new environment. This chair was selected with no less care than a cave-diver would spend choosing a system of air tanks. Let me walk you through the process.

First, we spent the better part of a day returning a recently purchased recliner that had turned into the Cujo of chairs in that it catapulted her across the room every time she pulled the lever to lower the footrest. So we returned the beast and turned our attention to the next generation of chair—deciding to forego the more testosterone-laden recliner for a good comfy armchair with a footrest, which seemed more benign. In Goldilocks fashion, "not too large and not too small—just right," we began our search. The ottoman had to be large enough to hold a tray while eating, watching the birds or television; had to easily glide along a carpeted floor (wheels) and be small enough to navigate around. The texture of the upholstery against thinning skin had to be soft, smooth and warm, and offer enough friction to prevent sliding around in it. This ruled out leather, and therefore, a large percentage of available stock. The back had to be high enough to provide head support, but not so tall or protruding that it felt like an airline seat. (Those of you under six feet tall know what I'm talking about.) Last, it needed to be attractive to her, ruling out funky plaids, Naugahyde and leopard print. Further, many of these factors had to be discerned by trial and error and the process of elimination, dealing with a woman who hailed forth from a generation taught NOT to speak their mind. (Add being psychic to the list of needed resources.) I know you're thinking this may be simple, but it wasn't, so finding the right one earned me a gold star for life.

Did I mention that it helps to be a diplomat?

Matters of the Heart

Fortunately, in another life stage, I'd worked in dispute resolution and mediated everything from barking dogs and pre-release sessions at a juvenile facility, to child/pet custody and property settlements. Those skills, along with both training and experience as a Victim Services Counselor—having supported victims of theft, violation, loss, etc.—should have, and ultimately did, serve me well in helping my mother as a victim. But the same skills we can apply flawlessly in non-emotional, less personal situations can sometimes fail to show up at all or arrive on the scene late when it comes to matters of the heart and our own families. We can stutter, succumb to old family patterns, make mistakes, and trip over our own egos to the point of acting downright stupid. It's one of the reasons doctors don't operate on their family and relatives make poor business partners. When emotions run high working with friends or family, old wounds can be re-exposed and fires fanned. It helps to have a few tools in your pocket that allow you get some distance, set personal boundaries, ask non-confrontational questions, and be supportive in the face of anger, grief, disorientation or territory disputes.

Letting Go

People are "one" with their possessions their memories, their dreams and their homes. Even those of us who do not have "clutter" issues, have trouble letting go of the non-tangibles that become paired with our treasures. Each interaction is fertile ground for applying some basic precepts borrowed from Eastern philosophies:

- Be fully present;

- Let emotions wash over you, but not become who you are;
- Ask each conflict what gift it offers;
- Offer compassion in place of judgment;
- Treat others as *they* would like to be treated, not as *you* would like to be treated.

This requires insight into what *we* bring to the process, some understanding of our own fears and foibles, and the ability to *not* engage in win/lose behaviors. One of the goals of this book is to offer tools and approaches to parting and reassessing with insight, humor and heart.

Incorporating my own experience with my mother, this book addresses the concerns voiced by hundreds of my students and clients. They run the gamut from combining households and moving into assisted living to addressing what we/they really *want* in this particular stage of life and the inevitable disputes over territory and ownership. Disputes can be as subtle as a difference of opinion. They don't have to be full blown donnybrooks.

Adult children often look back and realize they didn't take time to fully acknowledge or honor their parent's histories and that becomes a source of hurt and misunderstanding.

Crucial Process

We'll talk about the practical matters of how to go about such a project: how to get started, how to sort, how to make decisions to discard or recycle items and finding homes for those items and how to set up the new space. But my essential goal is provide a guide through a crucial process in a linear fashion, using non-linear tools. Sounds contradictory, doesn't it? Ultimately, however, we do our best work when we get the logarithmic power of merging the opposites of left and right brain, logic and intuition, mind and heart.

The Other End of the Journey

Over and over again, it is important to remind ourselves that we cannot use the template for earlier moves when moving our parents. When we were young and in our prime, most of us were still looking forward to expanding, just starting to accumulate and were for the most part healthy and surrounded by options and possibilities. Those of us facing the other end of the journey, moving into smaller places, divesting of material possessions, in preparation for the last half—and in some cases the last chapter—of our lives are engaged in a radically different process. Priorities shift and issues that were not even on the horizon in previous decades loom large. We can no longer steer around them or pretend they're not there. Methods of managing those realities and the incumbent emotions will be addressed.

> Helping a parent through the process means added baggage that we all carry with our parents, even though we love them dearly. When working with family, the emotional saboteur that has lurked behind the curtain of politeness in other encounters has a way of exploding like an angry teenager when we least expect it.

Since you are reading this book, chances are you were parented by or influenced in some way by the generation that went through the Great Depression. It is soul bending to know what some of our parents went through during this time. And it takes some understanding of this to really grasp why it's hard to throw out a piece of foil, why there are enough duplicate kitchen implements to equip several households, and why getting rid of almost anything taps into a rule-set foreign to those of us who never had to stand in line for sugar, make our underwear out of old flour sacks, or sell our tent or the tires off our car to buy food. Add to this the fact that they are looking toward transitioning and letting go of memory-laced and hard-won possessions, and the problem of releasing is magnified tenfold.

Geriatric Experience

In the mid-1970s, when I was young, naïve, idealistic, and fresh out of graduate school, I was hired to help develop and administer a statewide medical program. The focus of the program was to deliver hearing aids and related services to the state's elderly population on the basis of need. It was a job I had described in exquisite detail, as being my dream job a full year before it ever existed. When I was called for an interview, I was thrilled and I had no idea of how much I was about to learn. As an audiologist, I had experience with diagnostics and working in a medical clinic, but I had little political experience, and no real geriatric experience.

This was a controversial program, which I had to justify repeatedly to members of the legislature, and since I was so young, I encountered plenty of "good-ole-boys" who thought I needed to be taught a thing or two. They were right—and I did learn. In the way that only the very young have the luxury of believing, in my mind things were still black and white, right or wrong, and applicants were either qualified for the program or they weren't. Matters of hearing aids being stolen in the nursing homes or needing a hearing aid simply as a safety device to hear a car horn, the dog barking or the smoke alarm just didn't figure into my equation. On a trip to train local providers in the rules of the program, one of them asked if I'd ever visited a nursing home. My answer was no, and I didn't particularly want to. However, I was their passenger. Without warning, we arrived at the best facility the area had to offer. It smelled of Lysol, urine and medications, burning my nostrils, assaulting all of my senses and stabbing at my heart. Words fail miserably in describing the emotions that washed over me during that visit and I've never been the same. That experience continues to fuel my work.

Preserving Independence

Whatever we can do to preserve independence for our parents or ourselves, the resulting quality of life, autonomy, self-esteem and continuity with community are worth it. Even if you're not to the point of being concerned about some of these issues at present, we're all getting older—perhaps kicking and screaming all the way. The decisions we make now form the basis for the circumstances we (and our children) meet in the future. When there are no alternatives to nursing care, and it represents the best option, I hope this book will help guide aspects of that transition. Meanwhile, there are so many things that can be done along the way to adjust environments, relationships, communication and services. These are practical things, doable and affordable, and we owe it to ourselves to explore them.

Crucial Conversations

Much of our success hinges on how able we are to discern and articulate the crucial conversations—that naturally come up during this process, because every decision point shared with another person is an opportunity for conflict or collaboration. They arise over the most innocuous actions, as evidenced by an exchange that occurred between my mother and me during a visit to celebrate her 80th birthday. My sister and I had arrived on the scene from different coasts to help her celebrate, and also to deliver one of our gifts, which was to be available for a week to help her organize, decorate, and repair anything and everything. Aware that we might easily seem like steamrollers on a mission, we agreed to take it slowly, involve her in planning and executing, and to leave lots of time for fun in the form of bird-watching, movies, dinners out and sharing tales.

In the process of rearranging her bedroom for greater privacy and improving her sleep, we moved the bed and at her request and to her specifications installed two swing-arm reading lamps, one on each side of the bed. After measuring and reconfirming, I installed the fixtures. While I was tightening the last screws, she arrived on scene and announced, "That's not where I wanted them!" My inner pissed-off teenager was about to weigh in, which would have propelled us headlong down the win-lose path of verbal Armageddon I knew so well from my adolescence. Thank God, the adult in me took over and asked, "What doesn't work for you about this, and what would work better?" Knowing our past history, my sister waited in the wings, bracing for the explosion, but was stunned to witness instead an almost visible settling of Mom's feathers as she explained that now that she saw the lamp, she realized that she needed more room. No accusations about who was right or wrong came into play; no line-in-the-sand was drawn. Most important, she felt heard and validated, and later thanked me for being patient and willing to re-do something that had taken a lot of work—just to make her happy.

These types of events, handled with care, can change a relationship. Regardless of circumstance, people who feel they have been heard and acknowledged are more open to suggestions, feel less defensive and more appreciated, and have little need to fight the battle. Most important, they feel they still have options, the disappearance of which is one of the most devastating and disempowering aspects of old age.

Maintain Their Dignity

Over the years, I've spoken to many students and clients alike who have attempted to work with friends, relatives, or organizers with varying degrees of success, which depends largely on establishing and respecting boundaries. When working with a parent or friend, your job is to help categorize, ask the kinds of questions that will help with decisions, help keep them focused, energized and on task and offer suggestions and help with carrying out their decisions. Maintain their dignity at all costs. While it seems obvious, it is not your job to judge them or to coerce, bully, shame, or cajole them into getting rid of things *you* think are useless. Since they may be feeling extremely exposed (an emotion that can be expressed as defensiveness), one must be very conscious of the language being used. One client told his mother she needed to get rid of all her garbage, meaning, "Take out the trash."

In her vulnerable state of mind, she translated his literal use of the word "garbage" in a symbolic way—implying that all of her belongings (and therefore her life) were "garbage." Nor is it your job to make decisions based on what *you* perceive their needs to be (unless they are clearly too ill to participate) or to remove items they are unwilling to part with (because you think they won't notice). Don't treat them as children or otherwise embarrass them or cause them to feel helpless. Usually, we don't do such things consciously. Bullying can take the form of "the look," asking questions that imply superiority, or working long after their stamina has given out. It can be very covert and not recognized by the stronger party, only felt by the weaker. The caution to avoid inadvertent bullying would seem obvious, were it not for the stories shared about friendships lost, strained family relationships, and money wasted on hired helpers who violated these tenets through the mistaken idea that they were "helping."

What's Really of Worth?

This approach will give you tools for determining what's really of worth in your life or that of your parent. Every decision made in this process is focused on your parent's needs at this particular time in life and those that are likely to change in the near future. Realize from the start that this is a dynamic process and once into it, folks get more and more relaxed with the concept of letting go. The more control they have over the process, the greater the ownership and the less resistance. But it happens organically, inside the individual and is not something that can be forced. The more gentle and mindful the process, the greater the movement and benefit for both the individual and the caregiver, where one is involved.

> Above all, this is a heart-centered approach. It depends less on logic, what makes sense from the linear perspective, and what seems most rational from a dollars and cents point of view than what feels intuitively right.

There are many opportunities to apply pure logic, but even then it pays to listen to that little voice inside, perhaps to investigate further. If what seems obvious from a numbers position makes your gut tighten or your heart ache—investigate further, or wait. There's usually something going on. These signals may be arising from information you've yet to discover, or at least yet to understand. Ask questions of yourself or your parent to determine if there are unresolved issues, unspoken requests, fears, dreams or hurt feelings. When caring for an aging parent, our own fears can be the basis for decisions that run absolutely contrary to what they really need.

The essential difference with an older population is that we have to learn to listen with the "third ear" and our hearts, and practice recognizing the subtleties. Reading between the lines also helps. Yes, these are skills and attitudes helpful in any interaction, but more so when working with parents with whom we may have had a troubled history and/or those who are disoriented or angry at change and whose priorities are so radically different from our own because of age, income, mobility, etc.

Decisions

Many older people have begun to experience being treated as children, having decisions made for them by their own children who live at a faster pace and look at what's going to make their own lives easier. They have experienced going to physicians who are concerned only with saving their lives, not with the quality of the life that is saved, as Mom recently experienced after receiving her pacemaker. Still unable to breathe normally, one of the "risk indicators," listed in the Standard of Care information she received after the procedure, she called her doctor, only to be ignored. He reminded her that the pacemaker was simply to save her life and he had done that. He repeatedly discounted her fears about shortness of breath, greatly reduced stamina, and statements that she didn't want to "live like this." He'd done his job and wasn't concerned with the "frills." (Needless to say, she has new doctors who listen and are proactive.)

Indignities

Because they are living at a slower pace, there is an assumption made that their schedules don't matter as much that of someone who has a clock to watch. They have learned to suffer many indignities: reduced mobility results in their having to ask for help with tasks that used to be simple; reduced hearing results in their not understanding much of what is said, which in turn results in either social withdrawal or having to ask people to repeat and explain; reduced memory embarrasses them because they forget what's been said, can't remember if they took a medication, etc. The list goes on to include things like incontinence and a myriad of aches and pains. They begin to feel superfluous and believe they are burdens. When organizing for them, it's *soooo* easy to make decisions for them that make life harder, less fulfilling and less joyful.

Honoring

The goal here is to accommodate the need to move, organize, downsize, etc. while honoring quality of life. Their sense of belonging and integrity is essential. Determining and supporting those conditions and activities that bring joy and inclusiveness to life requires insight, skill, putting our own egos aside and a large dose of humor.

So let's get started...

2

A Sense of Place

Before digging into the details of how to go about the task at hand, I'd like to offer a look at the broader landscape we're trying to create once we arrive at our destination. Thinking of skipping this chapter because you want to focus on the nitty-gritty of your checklist and what to do next? This IS what you do next! It forms the underpinning of every decision to come. Think of it as the set design for the motion picture of the new life ahead, where we start thinking about the elements that will create the atmosphere that nurtures the script. These are the visions that let our spirits soar, even when our bodies are kicking their way through boxes and packing material. They give us energy as we paddle through the "swamp of despair" resulting from the thought of leaving the family home for whatever reason.

If visioning worked for Walt Disney (Capacchione, 2000), who always saw the finished product in his mind before he started, it can work for you. This is the glue that holds all the other pieces together and it's *the* essential piece to creating the space that will make it possible to adapt and thrive. More importantly, if this is being done for a parent, these are the ingredients that will foster his/her ability to emotionally settle-in to their new place. When that happens, they can start putting out feelers to new friends and activities beyond immediate family, thereby freeing everyone up for less dependency and greater freedom. Some of you probably do this visioning unconsciously, but I can say that once this is being done at a conscious level, the results are amazing. We'll talk more about this in Chapter Six, Creating the Experience You Want, but first, a story.

Inner Landscape

When Mom and I were digging through her papers—looking for warranties and other documents we needed to get her house listed—there, filed under "House," was a page torn from a magazine some 30 years ago.

Brown and fragile from age was a picture of a beautiful living room filled with color—peaches and greens, sunlight streaming through the windows, plants by the windows—the kind of room that makes you want to stop what you're doing and curl up on the couch, throw an afghan over your feet and read a book in the warm glow of contentment. I asked her about the picture and she said, "I've always wanted those colors in my house—a pretty couch, some reds and pinks..." Elegant, soft and feminine—it was the absolute antithesis of anything I ever thought my mother would want since I'd always seen her as an earthier soul, digging in her yard and concerned with practicalities. After all, we grew up with practical couches in colors that would tolerate muddy hands, juice spills, parakeet droppings and pet hair—in other words browns and tans except for one particularly ugly white vinyl thing inherited from a friend. I hated that couch.

I felt embarrassed for myself that I'd never known she's always wanted "soft and pretty," and saddened for her that she had just settled for the other. What a loss for both of us... As young girls, my sister and I were encouraged to buy neutrals: wearing colors that were soft and feminine, she told us, would diminish our ability to be taken seriously or to get "serious jobs." (Remember, it was the 1950s, and she was right!) I asked her why she'd never bought a pretty couch for herself, and her answer made me realize she'd resigned herself to never having pretty things—considered extravagant in depression years. Any couch would do; the small blue and brown rattan love-seat I gave her when I moved was the closest she ever came to having something that was just the least bit "frivolous!" I made it my mission to help create that feeling in her new apartment and the next week we bought the couch.

At first, she justified it as being the guest room bed. Since she'd moved into a smaller place, there was no longer an extra room, so she would need to make the second bedroom an office/guestroom combination. It would be OK to buy a couch for that room, because it was "necessary." While at the furniture store, she fell in love with a red micro-fiber couch, but it didn't come in a hide-a-bed, which is how she justified the purchase. The next store offered some similar options, but on sale in the back of the showroom was a sofa she would never have allowed herself to consider years ago. We discussed it and I watched as she went through the machinations of analysis and justifications that resulted in her getting a fabulous, shrimp pink hide-a-bed for her living room. For the first time in her life, she allowed herself to buy a "big" something with the emphasis on *her* enjoyment, rather than its being the most practical. I cannot describe the pure joy that erupted when the couch was delivered and placed in her living room. The old loveseat was moved to the guestroom, with the new rationalization that her guests could just sleep in the living room on the rare occasion she actually had an overnight guest and she could enjoy this beautiful couch every day.

Our physical environments are so much a reflection of our inner landscape. In Mom's choice of something that really made her happy, I could see a shift in her that meant she could relax a little with her life, let herself play a bit and give herself a gift. It's never too late and I want this stage of her life to be an "opening," not a closing. When you're going through belongings, be sure to notice what items, pictures and memories touch you and evoke that sense of place that transports you to the next level. Allow yourself and your parent the "luxury" of bringing those things along, even if it means leaving something more practical behind. Remember that 13th century poem:

> If of thy mortal goods thou art bereft,
> And from thy slender store two loaves along to thee are left,
> Sell one, and with the dole
> Buy hyacinths to feed thy soul.

A Greater Connection

Nowhere do I find this concept more important than in the work I do with my clients when called in to Feng Shui their homes. They call me because they want a greater connection with something they can't quite identify, but know it when it's there and feel a great sense of loss when it's absent. It's the quality of a place that speaks to the soul, the spirit of a place that whispers to the senses. And that is *not* created by mere attention to technical detail, practicality and function, conditions that characterize many of the places to which the elderly or infirm are relegated (or to which we relegate *ourselves*) when we are feeling pressed for funds, affection or lack the feeling that "we matter."

Sanctuary

Ever since humanity began living in shelters, we have been decorating our spaces, first with cave-drawings and later with drawings of caves, and other artwork of course. While we like to think of our species as unique, humans aren't the only ones to do this. There's a bird in Australia—the male Bower Bird—that decorates with such gusto and eye toward detail, it would put decorators to shame. Every little berry and feather is placed with precision. The females check around and find the most elaborately staged nest, and bingo! A match is made. It's so competitive that neighboring males will sneak in and throw things around while the owner is out gathering more supplies at the birdie Home Depot! Such is the nature of nest making and as every female Bower Bird knows, sticks alone do not make a home. Home, whether it's a cozy bungalow or a room in an Assisted Living Facility, should function as sanctuary: a place where we feel comfort, acceptance and safety, a place where we are creatively fertile—and one that motivates us to live our best lives.

> To thrive in a place, we must be emotionally engaged. If you're downsizing for yourself, or especially, if you're whittling down to the essentials for a parent moving into a few rooms, making decisions with the primary focus on utility and function could have devastating consequences.

The Medicine of Her Soul

The first thing I do when I move into a new place, after getting the bedroom and kitchen functional, is hang the artwork. Until I do, I feel displaced and out of focus. When moving Mom into her 1200 square feet of retirement living, everything was put in place within the first few days. Towels were folded nicely, the kitchen organized, meds and supplements stashed in easy to reach and remember places—even with an eye toward aesthetics. She had begun to make new acquaintances and had even met with her new heart specialist by the second week. An amazingly *efficient* move, really. But it wasn't until the artwork she'd collected over a lifetime of travel graced her walls that the twinkle came back into her eyes. I was dancing as fast as I could to get everything else in place so she could function safely and comfortably, and I ran out of steam and creative energy before I could hang the artwork. In retrospect, it would have been better to leave a few closets or boxes unpacked and to put the medicine of her soul in place. After basic needs have been met, it is the emotional connection to the place that begins to dampen the grief of leaving the old and the familiar behind. No amount of expert folding brings the same joy as your favorite painting!

Kidnapped By a Memory

It is so easy during this process to get tunnel vision—just "getting it done" because you have kids at home, a job, or husband or life! The left-brain takes over and functions like an economist, forgetting that there is little economy in ignoring emotions. We humans are awfully connected to places, even when we don't think so consciously. Our senses are engaged all of the time, even while we are navigating an unfamiliar street or putting away groceries. In every moment we are cataloging, and whammo! Right in the middle of something as mundane as going to the store we can be kidnapped by a memory that takes us to another place and time.

Once as I was browsing in an antique store in Austin, Texas, I caught a whiff of something that transported me back in time to a place with sea breezes, spices and the scent of furniture oil. Instantly, *I am there*—not like I was seeing it in the "mind's eye," but physically on that spot. The salty breeze on my skin! The smell of cumin and Harissa peppers! I am disoriented—and hear the Muslim call to prayer. Aware of old wood under my fingertips—I am running my hands over an old marriage chest, hand-painted and oiled to protect it against the ravages of the 100 plus years since it was crafted. When the memory circuits of my brain finally identified it, I realized I was standing in a shop on a hilltop in Sidi Bou Said, Tunisia, a peninsula artist colony surrounded by the azure blue of the Mediterranean. In a heartbeat a whiff of oil used for thousands of years to protect wood had propelled me back to a place imprinted in my soul over twenty years ago. This one sense, this body memory, had re-connected me to the energetic *field* of a place where I'd spent only thirty minutes a lifetime ago. Imagine the connections we form living in a place where we have raised kids, baked pies, bandaged skinned knees, experienced love and loss, joys and disappointments.

Trappings

Place—its smells, sounds, images and feelings—has the ability to engulf us in comfort, take us back in time or throw us to the wolves. In the military or any institution whose purpose it is to mold all minds into one disciplined endeavor, the first element removed is the freedom to personalize one's space and one's appearance, thereby cutting all ties with your old self. After entering the navy, my son (and every other enlistee), sent the last vestige of his identity home in a box containing the pants, shirt, belt and underwear he'd worn to his swearing in, along with his wallet and ID. Ridding us of our trappings creates anonymity, leaves us without the feeling of roots, disorganizes our habits and thought patterns and we lose our bearings. The highest mortality in nursing homes comes within the first six months—the adjustment period for being away from one's home, family, belongings and community.

Corporations that house their employees in de-personalized cubicles have an extremely high turnover as people feel a lack of connection and loyalty—they feel less valued. Being humans, our connection to our environment imparts a sense of control over our life and its possibilities. It echoes where we have been and can mentor us into becoming who we want to be. It's no wonder we can feel so undone by a move and why transporting even a minimum of treasures that carry scent, tactile memory and our history serve as a reference point from which to create a new life. Without them we feel adrift, displaced.

> Like the yeast culture used as the "starter" for a fresh batch of sourdough bread, even a few of our belongings brought to a sterile new environment can act as the culture from which to grow a new life.

When doing the selecting and discarding for your parent, here's a word of warning: don't make the mistake of thinking that *you* know what these items are. *Ask!* To throw out things because we think they won't know is a psychic violation that transcends the obvious. Crossing that threshold can create a crisis of trust that seeps into other areas. There is a form of arrogance to this type of unilateral decision-making (except when there is medical necessity and your parent is truly non compos) or bullying that does great damage. Sometimes we simply get our signals crossed and inadvertently assume we are helping, until it's discovered that we threw out or moved something perceived as valuable. Regaining the trust that gives us the latitude to move ahead can take months.

With age comes a great deal of fear associated with losing control or access to our belongings, and no matter how much you love and think you know someone, it's a mistake to assume it's OK to discard or rearrange certain things. On the other hand, discussing, sharing, and setting respectful boundaries engender trust, healing and relationship building. The gift in this process is that you may actually have a deeper relationship with your parent than ever before.

The goal is to create or re-create a place that engages mind, body and spirit. The body is taken care of by finding living space that is safe and easy to navigate. It should offer proximity to medical care and support activities like grocery shopping, pharmacy visits, and everyday maintenance. So when you're doing your planning, consider simultaneously how to keep the other connections intact. When my sister and I were packing Mom's house in stages over a six-week period, we knew how stressful it would be to live in disarray. Therefore, it was that much more important to keep her books for crossword puzzles, reading, etc., accessible—and neither moved nor packed prematurely. On the other end, those were the things that came out and were put in place first.

Matters of spirit were a little harder to manage, because moving is such a disruptive event and because many of the things that made her happy were being left behind. It's mighty hard to pack the bird population of south Louisiana and move it 500 miles west, so we had to settle for keeping all the bird feeding going until the absolute last moment and I do mean we were feeding birds right up until the movers pulled away. She was grieving over "abandoning" her birds, so it was helpful that her neighbors took over some of the feeders. We also took a few of the feeders with us, and they were filled at her new place by the end of the second day. The fact that a pair of house finches was seen noshing on a fresh supply of black oil sunflower seeds by the end of that day brought more comfort and joy than having her kitchen organized. When we have some soul connection in place, it's easier to tolerate other inconveniences. Without some glimmer of joy, it's easy to emotionally shut down and barricade ourselves against further disappointment and disruptions.

Now's the time to sit and talk a few minutes with your mom or dad and fantasize over what would be wonderful to have in the "new place." This took a little doing with Mom. Initially, she was too overwhelmed with the details of getting packed and disconnected from her home. Here are some ideas to help that process along:

- Make a pot of tea or coffee, have a snack and play a little *what-if* game: if you could have any color you wanted, what would it be?

- Cut dream pictures out of magazines! Even if you can't completely redecorate, old things can be used in new ways so that it all feels *new*.

This creative time is magical in that it inspires a vision of moving toward, instead of moving away, from something. It's an instant mood booster and lets you feel you're doing this together.

Summary and Major Points

1. Creating a sense of place in your parents' new home will foster their ability to emotionally settle in.
2. Our physical environment is a reflection of our inner landscape and must engage mind, body and spirit.
3. Avoid making unilateral choices about what is valuable for your parent.
4. Discussing, sharing, and setting respectful boundaries engender trust, healing and relationship building.
5. Fantasizing about how we want the new place to look and feel creates a sense of moving toward, instead of away, from something.

Suggested Activities

These activities can be done in a number of ways. Your parents might like to do these alone or with you as a shared way of really paying attention to the sensations that represent home as it is and what they would like to re-create or change at the new place. If your parents are unable to participate, these activities can help you, their helper, identify sights, sounds and aromas that might be triggers to help them feel more "at home" elsewhere.

1. Take a moment of quiet time, close your eyes and mentally walk through their home.

- What is the image, aroma, or sound that first comes to mind?

- Are there one or two special things that capture this essence of home?

- If you could only take three things with you to a new place (other than spouse or other family members) what would they be?

2. Gather some magazines (decorating, travel, sports, financial) and over tea or coffee tear out pictures of "what grabs you." Do it on impulse, don't think it through. Grab any image that speaks to you without analyzing it.

3. Cut the pictures out and make a dream board. You can learn a lot about yourself and your parents from this carefree activity. Remember the couch!

3

Getting Started

Without a doubt, each of us comes to the point of moving our parents—or ourselves, from a different vantage point. When I moved back to Texas from West Virginia, I'd made very deliberate choices about my future. The move to West Virginia was purely intuitive and I really just followed my instincts, knowing they have never led me astray—though sometimes the path has been circuitous! The move back, however, was deliberate in every aspect. I'd looked at several places I've loved visiting, but Central Texas is my true spiritual home. For those of you moving by choice to your Dream retirement, give thanks! You have options and this book will help you fine-tune them.

For our parents, the move may have come about differently. For Mom, thoughts of moving were never on the horizon until she began toppling over while doing yard work. Her knees were giving her trouble and it looked like digging up weeds, mowing the grass and hiking in New Mexico may have to drop by the wayside (at 82)! Breathing had become labored as she was diagnosed with a slight case of emphysema from living with a chain-smoker under the toxic skies of petrochemical and bauxite plants, but even that couldn't keep her down. Her knees and breathing problems were not, however, the issues. It seems that the passing out was related to the fact that her heart rate would drop perilously low and she would faint, at which point it would pick up and she'd perk up. She had the pacemaker inserted, and we wrongly assumed it would remedy most of the fatigue. The doctor from hell said the pacemaker was to save her life, which he had done and anything else was essentially irrelevant. Even family intervention resulted only in the doctor chastising my mother for siccing her daughters on him. He never adjusted the pacemaker.

We realized that this sort of brusque and heartless medical care had become routine for her in Lake Charles, so something had to be done. The final blow for her was the double onslaught of hurricanes Rita and Katrina, which spared her home but not the bird population so dear to her heart.

We thought her move to Texas would allow for greater independence because she wouldn't have the overhead of caring for house, birds and yard. We knew, with family close, she would receive better medical care. We reasoned that the air quality and reduced humidity would help with breathing and energy levels. But what would she look forward to? What would replace the grumbling, yet loving care of her yard, those "pesky" birds that needed feeding three times a day, and "those damn squirrels" she threw shoes at? All of this brings us to this point:

> Moving "away from" is not enough. We must know what we are moving toward.

So if you're just itching to start cleaning out and packing things, hold on a second and consider where you're going. What do you want the end product to be? In fact, spend some time really ferreting out what you want to impact by moving. Are you seeking:

- A simpler, more authentic lifestyle?
- A more manageable house or smaller footprint?
- Closer connections to family?
- Opportunity to travel?
- Time and space to pursue creative pursuits?
- Better health care?
- A space that offers improved mobility?
- A location for your parent to live out their final years?
- A retirement lifestyle?
- A new challenge or business?

In the act of relocating, sometimes we become so focused on leaving our current situation (or finding a place for Mom and Dad to live out their final years) that we get caught up in the mechanics of the move only to find ourselves in a space that suits us less well than the one from which we'd moved. If that's true, it's because we have failed to be mindful of what it is we really want. We have been in response mode instead of creation mode.

Changing Spaces

Every move into a new space, or reorganization of an existing one, starts with the knowledge that something is changing or needs to change. How we feel about change depends in part on whether we planned it or are responding to circumstances that make change necessary, and how much thought has been given to what we want the destination to look like. Ever found yourself driving along on autopilot, and then looking up in amazement, wondering how you got there? Worse yet, trying to remember where you were going in the first place? Starting any project without visualizing your goal is fraught with unanticipated obstacles, disappointments, and losing our way.

Consider the home of Eleanor, a Parkinson's client, where a friend's efforts to create more space in the bedroom resulted in clogging passageways elsewhere, making the home nearly impassable. Her unsteady gait and need to stabilize with broad sideways, jerky steps required unobstructed pathways and plenty of space to maneuver. Failure to look at the bedroom project holistically resulted in making her home unsafe for her to move around in and blocked essential escape routes in case of an emergency.

In another instance—in an AIDS support center offering community and comfort for patients and their families—rooms were painted muddy red and filled with donated artwork of disjointed bodies. Lack of awareness about the symbolism of the artwork and the psychological and physiological impact of the dirty-blood-colored walls created the opposite of the desired effect.

Elsewhere, there are nursing home interiors painted in a depressing grey-beige, a color that creates an overall feeling of dinginess and despair. Such surroundings counteract efforts to keep patients physically healthy by ignoring the impact of color and ambience on emotional well-being.

In the case of moving or reconfiguring an existing space, proceeding forward without giving deep attention to what we want life to look like on the other end can be even more catastrophic. Sometimes we look up and wonder why we're doing this or how we got to this point. It's probably not early Alzheimer's. Sometimes our mental circuits are just overloaded—or we're simply not paying attention to what matters most. But chances are, you may not have an organized approach to integrating all of the factors to be considered. How often do we find we've been living life that way? It's a common problem encountered in many of life's transitions.

Choices

Years ago, my job at an employment outplacement firm was to train and counsel groups of recently *riffed* employees. Riffs or large scale "reductions in force," common in high tech, always leave a trail of angry, confused and frightened out-of-work people in their wake. In the context of these work-shops, I found that most individuals tended to go after the same type of job they'd just left, because it was what they'd always done, but not necessarily what they wanted or liked to do.

We can live on autopilot for years in the same job or the same house, complaining about the same things, yet never taking time to question or rethink our options. In the resume writing part of these workshops I always asked, "So, what is it you *choose* to do?" It's a question that made even the most successful executive quake. "Well, this (work) is what I've always done, what I'm trained to do—I've never really thought about what I *want* to do. I just need to make money and this is how I've always done it."

When given the opportunity to see the RIF as a chance to define what they might actually *like*, or to find or create a position that would be fulfilling, not just functional in terms of income, they began to see possibilities. With possibilities came excitement and renewed interest in the quest. Anger dissipated, confusion became insight, and the search for a new "job" became an opportunity to make choices and to live life differently—perhaps reducing stress and re-evaluating. It didn't happen overnight and it didn't remove the necessity of finding a new job. What it did do was offer the real potential of living more authentically, and actively crafting a life in which they could become emotionally engaged and more satisfied.

This story has implications for relocating. Even if we are riffed—ousted from our current lifestyle against our conscious will—we also have a chance to ask, "What do I want?" It's not fair to answer with "three bedrooms, two baths!" That's just function, and we're going after something more.

> "As we age, we tend to focus more on "purpose, intrinsic motivation, and meaning."
> —Daniel Pink

These are the things we might have neglected when we were on the fast track to success and raising our 2.5 kids. Psychologist David Wolfe, writing about older adults in *Ageless Marketing* (2006), states "...perceptions of self and the world about them tend to be strongly influenced by contextual circumstances." Life becomes more about meaning—who we are in the context of community and being emotionally engaged with our environments. So, these moves really can be about starting a new phase, consciously focused on what will make life meaningful and purpose-driven. The second half of life offers the opportunity to refashion our lives and express creativity we had little time for or interest in when we were younger.

One turning-sixty professional couple opted to leave Washington D.C., where one had worked for the State Department and the other was a Ph.D. trainer in the field of psychology. Seeking a challenge where they would both learn something new, continue to be near family in a smaller community, get back to the land and real physical work, and create a self-sustaining lifestyle, they chose to buy an old farm. They decided to raise cattle and live in a small, but eclectic and diverse community where they could contribute at a grass roots level. By consciously choosing every aspect of their life they constructed a new second-half filled with family, community ties, and hard but satisfying work. They bridged the old lifestyle to the new one by commuting for a couple of years until they got the farm up and running.

Another couple relocated to a small town they had called home over a decade ago in order to be nearer their grandchildren, saying good-bye to the extremely lucrative real estate market in Phoenix. After re-building a client base, they are now designing a way to bridge the transition from the hectic pace of selling real estate to travel, writing and photography. These conscious proactive decisions are made possible by having a system to analyze all of the factors.

So, what do we choose? And why is it so difficult to come up with the answers to that question? In looking back at how we were reared, four reasons come to mind and they relate to mindset and the rules we were taught or absorbed in our childhoods. As you read through these, they might offer some insights into why it is so difficult to get our parents to talk about what would really make them happy during the next stage and thus solve the mystery behind their attachment to possessions which, to us, have little value.

As generations born on opposite ends of World War II and the Depression, we represent radically different paradigms. The post WWII generation is the first to straddle that gap which places one foot in depression era mind-set and the other balanced on the dualistic concepts of consumerism and spiritual consciousness. To get an idea of why it is so hard for us (and especially our parents) to think in terms of what we want for ourselves, we have only to examine some of the rules and values our parents lived by and with all good intentions, passed on to us, their children.

1. **Be grateful for what you have (i.e., it's sinful to want more).** Regardless of age, and sometimes because of it—we are still operating from what Carolyn Myss (*Anatomy of the Spirit*, 1996) might term "tribal rules," the oft-unspoken; yet hard-wired rules handed down through generations, defining attitudes ranging from sexuality to aspirations. Constructed from the fall-out of depression era thinking (survival is tough—it's selfish to think of what you want—be grateful you have food on the table, don't ask for happiness—there are starving people everywhere...) we were taught not to "want." As a post WWII baby-turned-adult, I know I am not alone in this experience. Our parents learned the survival tools of hard work, conservation of resources, stoicism, and the philosophy of "don't ask/don't tell." What worked for them during the depression is a contrary force in today's consumerist world.

No one would suggest that conservation of resources at both a personal and a global level is not worthwhile, but in depression era vernacular that meant saving every last piece of foil, plastic bag, piece of string and broken implement. It meant being happy with what you have, and not allowing yourself to want something better or even different. Gratitude became synonymous with sacrifice and some wants were considered downright sinful. My mother tells the story of her mother (my sweet, frail, wouldn't hurt a fly, church-going grandmother...) chasing her around the cotton patch with a stick because Mom (then a teenager) wanted a "store-bought" brassiere! Her *wanting* was considered not only greedy, but sinful as well!

This thought-form has contributed to debilitating clutter in our current culture of easy acquisition, reduced shelf life, and built in obsolescence. It also provides the ammunition for an internal war, as we fall over our possessions and still are no closer to knowing what we want. When it becomes time to move for our parents, there can be a real void of knowing what would be optimum, because they've habituated to what "is," and are imprisoned by the very possessions and ideas that supported them long ago. As their children, we can be similarly boxed in by our guilt over wanting a different reality that we struggle to define. Finally, we *also* have possessions we "should" feel guilty about both having (greed) and throwing away (wasteful).

2. Work before pleasure. Next, there is the Calvinistic thinking characterized by work before play, and hard work being the key to progress and therefore well-being and salvation. (Disclaimer: I am *not* condemning hard work.) This approach also served the depression era generation exquisitely, so became more deeply justified. It's not just the Christian/western religions that hold that standard. Buddhism also talks about life being filled with suffering and admonitions to learn to love what you have.

I may be oversimplifying here, but we have all been brought up with these fundamentals in our culture. Even if we didn't grow up going to weekly prayer meeting, reading scripture or saying *Hail Marys*, the rule was "work hard, play later." The post-war generation added, "if it feels good, do it," and we're a little schizophrenic about it, having been schooled in relegating pleasure to the back burner. If we had time to play, we then had to contend with the guilt built in to #1 (Be grateful for what you have). As another tribal rule, it is so deeply rooted that it permeates life without being spoken.

We learned that following these cultural rules resulted in approval, and not abiding by them carried stiff consequences of rejection. The practice of "shunning" in Amish culture represents one extreme of not playing by the rules. By the time we are adults, we've been thoroughly indoctrinated and have become so good at adapting and responding that we have no idea of how to start the process of investigating what we want, even if we can convince ourselves it's OK to ask. The problem here is that we now know that our attitudes and emotions about life can and do impact the reality we create. Keeping ourselves from joy and anticipation actually places a roadblock to the very things we think we will "earn" by concentrating on "all work and no play." We create our best lives through enjoyment, excitement and gratitude combined with doing the work we *love*.

In the depression, loving your work was not part of the equation. You got a job and you kept it until you got the gold watch. When you retired, the reward for your twenty years of loyalty was the pension. The current economy, high-tech market and shifting sands of industry have made long-term security a thing of the past, and pensions unreliable as corporations take Chapter 11. Our current quest for balance in work and pleasure results in some internal conflict, but it is also creating a new life paradigm.

3. Don't get excited—it might not happen. Third is the warning we learned at our parent's knee, lovingly taught as a way of protecting us from disappointment, "Now don't get too excited—you know it might not happen, and we don't want you to be disappointed!" Nearly everyone I know identifies with this, so I think it must be pretty universal. Remember when, as a kid, you'd get so jazzed about something you hoped for? Nearly always, our excitement was followed by an adult admonishing us to "not get so excited." Our current understanding of how we attract or impact our reality tells us just the opposite. We MUST be able to visualize it, be excited about it to manifest it. Still, it is a life-lesson so deeply embedded it takes conscious languaging and thought reframing to re-train ourselves. More on that process in Chapter Six.

4. Well, I know what I DON'T want. Finally, being asked, "What do you want?" can be a little like being thrown into the middle of the sea without a raft or a map. It's overwhelming, too broad a question, and the answer defined by context. The first volley of answers might include: "shark repellant—no, no make that a raft!" and "oh yeah—which direction is land?" Demands for water and food might follow, with demands for sunscreen, a paddle, and an EPIRB (emergency position-indicating radio beacon). The answer depends on where we are on the continuum from survival to perfection; what category we're talking about and how soon we want whatever it is. So it helps to have a structure or context in which to frame the question and therefore the answer(s).

To be able to answer the question, "What do you want?" one needs a structure, something to identify the elements or the categories of the project. And the project is "life," (not just changing houses). We've got this body, and this life, and we've been toddling around more or less without a map, and now we've arrived at a destination, which may or may not be of our active choosing. The operative word here is *active,* because we still choose in every moment. However, more often than not the choice is made through default. Think of it as inheriting a car... Now that we've got it, *is it what we would have chosen had we known we could choose?* Does it work? What's not working?

So we begin to think about systems, and there are some rules about the way things work. We're not sure what they are, but we know there is bound to be some logic involved and we have an owner's manual, to use the car analogy. We dig in: the car runs fine, but the reverse-lights aren't working. What's the problem? This literally happened to me a few months ago, so I started what amounts to a systems analysis, using the manual as a starting place in an effort to avoid a huge repair bill that would result if I took it to the dealership and let them "trouble shoot" at $96/hour. Electrical, I thought—wiring, light bulbs, etc. Nothing there. Not the transmission—it goes into reverse just fine. Not bulbs—they'd been checked. Fuses! That's it! Nope—fuses fine. Finally, having eliminated all of those, I took it to the shop and found it was a tiny switch (not mentioned in the manual but positioned on the transmission chassis) that sends the message to the reverse-lights to turn on. So the systems were defined, but to the uninitiated (me), there was no information about how these two systems interacted or communicated to give me reverse lights. At least there was an actual part that made the connection. It's not so straightforward in life, and goodness knows there are plenty of chances for fouled communication.

Why are we talking about cars? Because life, too, is a constellation system: **Physical** (the body, house, car, and belongings), **Mental** (thoughts, abilities, aptitudes, ideas, and intentions) and **Spiritual** (emotions, wisdom, character, intuition, connections).

To complicate matters, they're all integrated, so that if changes occur in one, the others are impacted. The goals we set for our professional life impact health, family and social life just as our social life can impact health, professional life and family. Moving and reorganizing are filled with variables so numerous it's dizzying. Every decision impacts every other decision, like a crossword puzzle—just changing a vowel can create order or chaos. We're back to doing a systems analysis—looking at priorities and determining what works.

One approach is to look at our needs and prioritize them. Abraham Maslow (1908–1970), known for his work in humanistic psychology and theories of self-actualization, created the now famous **hierarchy of needs**. Working with monkeys, he noticed that some needs are more critical than others. He parleyed this observation into needs ranging from *Deficit needs* (water, air, food and sex), the lack of which, according to Maslow, could kill you, to physiological needs, safety and security, love and belonging, self-actualization, and finally, the transcended state.

Mona Lisa Schultz in her book, *The New Feminine Brain* (1998), looks at the effects of any traumatic sense of loss. Such losses can include loss of community and affection in general. She notes that they can result in enormous hormonal and other chemical changes in the body. The results often include depression, exhaustion, and a compromised immune system, leaving us feeling bereft and isolated even from our own coping mechanisms.

Roger Fisher and William Ury, in their book *Getting to Yes: Negotiating Agreement Without Giving In* (1981) talk about identifying interests in the process of negotiation. They state the "most powerful interests are basic human needs," another way of stating Maslow's theory. They offer the following list of needs: *security, economic well-being, a sense of belonging, recognition* and *control over one's life.*

As universal as these classifications are, they lack the specificity that allows us to break life down into the manageable, concrete parts that help us make plans and decisions about the very physical act of relocating and fine-tuning our lives.

So What Does Work?

If we had been provided with an owner's manual for constructing a life that works, it might look like the one that came through some of the Eastern philosophies, which have long recognized that everything is connected. It's less linear, more collaborative, encompasses all the components of Maslow's hierarchy and uses terminology we understand at the practical level, while offering tools that work at the symbolical level—the language of the soul. By blending the physical, psychological and spiritual aspects of life, it provides a foundation that recognizes the interdependency of the systems, while giving us both common sense guidelines and room to engage the spirit. The approach I've used in private life and with my clients for the last decade is borrowed from the spiritual eastern philosophy of Feng Shui, but adapted for a western mind-set. It embraces the sciences of ergonomics, Quantum Physics and psychology. Although we are all unique, we do the *same types of things* in unique ways.

For the uninitiated, this ancient system originated nearly 10,000 years ago as a science of observation, the goal of which was to maximize a farmer's ability to thrive by orchestrating the planting of crops and orienting the home in accordance with observed weather patterns and natural formations. Over thousands of years, it evolved into a comprehensive model that gives us the means to remove obstacles and harmonize our environments. It hinges on the understanding that man and his environment are one and that our physical environment is a metaphor for how we live life.

> "We shape our dwellings, and afterwards, our dwellings shape us."
>
> —Winston Churchill

When Churchill made that statement, he echoed what philosophers (Aristotle), mathematicians (Fibonacci), psychiatrists (Karl Jung), and architects (Hindertwasser, and Clare Cooper Marcus in her book *House as a Mirror of Self*, 1995) continued to rediscover in seemingly divergent disciplines: that the space in which we live dramatically influences how life evolves in every category from health to intimate relationships.

The wisdom of this practice continues to be relevant because the ancient masters knew intuitively what science has only recently been able to explain and document. Feng Shui, which literally translated means "wind" and "water," referring both literally and figuratively to the elements in our lives, gives us a method to interact with the vibrational energy that connects all things. Thought, action and form are connected and interdependent in this field of ambient potential. Change one variable, and everything else responds. In addition to the ergonomic principles, much of the strength of this approach derives from the requirement that we become clear about our intentions in living each of nine separate, but related aspects of life. These *Life Domains are:*

- Health/Unity/Wholeness;

- Career and how we fill our time (activities);

- Knowledge (Wisdom) and Spirituality;

- Family and New Beginnings;

- Wealth and Manifestation (Finances);

- Reputation and Extensions into Community;

- Relationship (spouse/significant other);

- Creativity and Vision of the future;

- Travel and Benefactors.

A Holistic System

When we move, every aspect of life is both impacted by the move and impacts the process. This system is at once concrete, leaves no stone unturned and simultaneously acknowledges mind, body, and spirit. In short, it is a holistic system that meets all of our needs. If we enter the process by considering each of these factors, we simultaneously create for ourselves a picture of the larger landscape: the big picture of how we want our lives to unfold. At a macro level, we get rid of what doesn't support us. By creating the opportunity for a smoother and less stressful move, we are less apt to be blind-sided and will feel honored in the process of creating a life that really works.

> "The best prescription for these modern maladies may be to approach one's own life in a contextual big-picture fashion—to distinguish what really matters and what merely annoys."
> —Daniel Pink

Soul-Searching

We are asked to do some soul-searching to discover what our heart's desires (including thoughts, emotions and attitudes) are in each of these nine life categories. That's the starting point, and while it might seem ethereal, I guarantee it is a practical approach to ultimately reaching goals. For the purposes of this book, the goals are:

- To make the move to a new living situation (or adaptation of the current one) the best possible in all respects; and

- To offer the means to create a life that is supportive at every level.

It's a system that works.

Let's look at what's involved in each of these domains and at least a few of the issues that pop up in each. This is the basis for beginning to think about this move as something other than boxes, moving vans and hassle. It's the opportunity to think about what we really want in each area. What would make the heart sing? What's optimum? Where's the primary focus?

In absolutely concrete terms, knowing the choices in each of these domains will help define:

- Where we want to be;

- What we take with us on the journey;

- How we pack;

- How we organize and settle in at the other end.

A bit of time given to this process will save you TIME, MONEY and FRUSTRATION at both ends of the process. It will help create not only a supportive environment, but also a process that builds relationship and collaboration.

The Nine Life Domains Explained

HEALTH

This includes any and all issues that impact health and the ability to feel the best in whatever the circumstances might be. Even in cases where the ideal is not possible, optimization is.

While this category looks at physical and medical requirements, it also addresses ancillary systems that support a general sense of well-being and sense of being cared for. It includes attention to documents, contacts and schedules. Not only do these details relate to physical necessity, just knowing that critical documents are accessible is a contributing factor in reducing anxiety and feeling protected and prepared.

In practical terms, attending to things like large print on medication bottles and tops that can be opened with arthritic hands makes the difference in the comfort level in self-care and whether medications are taken at all. Sometimes, attention to these details can make a difference in remaining in one's own home versus moving to assisted living or a nursing home.

When I was the Director of a Hearing Aid Program for the Department of Human Resources, one of the issues that came up repeatedly was the importance of a hearing aid in allowing someone to remain in their home—even when the loss was so profound that understanding speech was out of the question. The ability to hear the phone, a knock on the door, or a fire alarm is also critical to safety and independence.

CAREER and ACTIVITIES

This domain is not just about work, but about what a person does with his/her time in the world. If one is working, it certainly includes a literal career, but could also refer to hobbies, volunteer work, and the opportunities that come to us via the "river of life." Consider what activities bring meaning to life and whether those will be supported or interrupted by the move.

When I lived in West Virginia near my sister, we were constantly talking about how we could get our mother to move nearer to us. We wanted to be closer to help her with any health matters and for her to more easily be involved in family gatherings. Since airline travel had become such a problem for her that she preferred a 30-hour bus ride, having her live closer seemed like a good idea at the time. She kept telling us she was too old to get reconnected to a new community, that she couldn't be away from her bird watching and volunteer work. We, of course, thought that with our help she could recreate these connections elsewhere. That opinion changed when I went birding with her in the marshlands around Lake Charles and experienced first hand her joy and total shift of disposition when she was with her birds. The vibrancy, curiosity and purpose that I'd remembered from earlier days re-emerged. Only when hurricane Katrina destroyed these bird-friendly ecosystems (and it will take decades—if ever—to reclaim them), did she consider a move.

Another day, I went with her to meet the staff at an elementary school where she volunteered in the library. As a retired reference and children's room librarian, she was an invaluable resource to this poorly funded school, but more importantly, everyone there treated her like family. They hugged her and let her know how important her work was, gave her homemade rolls from the cafeteria, and in all ways reaffirmed her importance. It kept her physically active, emotionally supported and spiritually connected. We stopped suggesting that she move, unless it became a physical imperative. That time has now come and we are in the process of finding a way to replace those treasured connections.

In practical terms, it is important to be near activities that bring meaning to everyday life and having the means of accessing these. How close is the nearest quilting shop, bird sanctuary, library, golf course? If your parent is an artist, where will he or she paint?

KNOWLEDGE and SPIRITUALITY

This domain addresses matters of the spirit, which might include religion, but is not limited to that. It represents the ability to make wise decisions and take action. This area is less about academic matters and more about being able to bring all of the life experiences and knowledge one has gathered into the wisdom of making decisions, mentoring, and feeling connected to life source energy. It might include access to classes, community education, a library and other venues to keep mentally and spiritually active.

Although it's not about religion, many people access their spirituality through religious activities. Therefore retaining connections to a supportive religious or spiritual community or finding a new one is important. Spirituality is a very individual matter and doesn't always include outside activities, but does pertain to whether people feel connected to a source of inspiration, their own inner guidance system and whether they trust themselves and others to provide for their wellbeing.

In practical terms, this could relate to privacy, access to churches, meditation groups and activities that nurture the spirit, and the respect afforded an individual's intuitive sense of what they need. In other words, we must listen with a respectful heart and be able to read between the lines to hear what the spirit is whispering.

FAMILY

This domain includes, but is not limited to, biological family. It can include members of the community or social group that feel like family and would want to be intimately involved in this person's life. As families have become more mobile, it is increasingly unusual to find parents and children living in the same communities. Many senior moves take place specifically to create proximity to children, but fail to consider the loss of the family of friendships that have been created and that will be lost upon moving.

Later in life, friendships are harder to re-create and attitudes are more deeply entrenched. Differences in political, spiritual or religious affiliations become important considerations when one becomes less mobile. After moving into a comfortable retirement community, one client reported feeling as though she'd moved to Mars, because the political climate was so alien to her. Another lamented the loss of younger contacts and the fact that conversations centered on ailments and loss.

In practical terms, does the place under consideration offer a philosophical match and the potential for supportive family or friendship groups? Is there any family near? Have there been any conversations regarding the disposition of belongings? What are their feelings about receiving support from family?

FINANCIAL AFFAIRS

This domain includes any and all matters relating to fiscal responsibility and the activities needed to maintain finances. Prosperity is also about feeling in control of the life we want to create for ourselves, and feeling that resources are available to accomplish that goal. This is very much tied to our essential outlook on life and whether it is one of fear and lack, or one of possibility and abundance.

In practical terms, this addresses the allocation of resources, the physical location of documents, legal papers such as Power of Attorney, and access to resources in the case of emergency. New bank accounts, service accounts, telephone connections, etc. assume a higher emotional priority when the move takes one away from family and friends and a higher safety priority where health issues are present.

EXTENSIONS INTO COMMUNITY

In the discipline of Feng Shui this is usually referred to as Fame, which involves issues of character, reputation and how one relates to community. It also addresses community interface and how those around us view us— as helpful, reliable, generous, miserly, dependant, etc. Whether right sizing or moving into a retirement community, this consideration would involve whether there are avenues for continuing to be recognized for contributions or opportunities for leadership, teaching, mentoring, or sharing of skills and resources.

In practical terms, continuity between how our parents were known in their community and the contributions they would like to make in their new community is important for well-being. We have to consider both knowledge and items they will take with them to support that connection and what resources need to be contacted to assist with this continuity. I've had several clients who rated taking along their games as a higher priority than usual, because they represented a way to connect to new friends.

RELATIONSHIP (Self and Intimates)

This domain involves one's spouse or any person with whom one is sharing an emotionally close relationship. It could even be a business partnership or housemate with whom deeply personal information is shared.

Because external issues mirror internal issues, at the core of this life domain is one's relationship to self. If you're helping a parent move and issues of trust and abandonment come up, they are usually less about the external relationship and more about how those issues have been handled internally with self. Furthermore, age and illness can conspire to conjure up monsters and foreboding wherever or whenever personal space is eroded or changed.

In practical terms, how can we support our relationship with partner, parent or ourselves during this stressful event? If our parent and his/her spouse are living apart, how is this likely to affect them? What is the fall-out for the family? How does one feel about self in this new context and what support systems are in place to help with the transition?

CHILDREN, FUTURE and CREATIVITY

This domain was addressed a bit under family, so we'll focus on the issue of future, and at later stages of life, the future can be uncertain. As younger people, the future seemed to spread out ahead of us like a Kansas wheat field: no end in sight. A lot of the big things we've looked forward to have already been done—family, career, and ownership. Now there might be travel, time to read and learn just for the fun of it, spiritual discovery, golf, or volunteering. Explore consciously the things most enjoyed and make every effort to accommodate those pleasures in the new place.

In practical terms, will hobbies and activities change, and if so what will be discarded or taken? What will change and how can we prepare for a smooth transition? In Mom's case, most of her gardening equipment went to a grandson and bird feeders went to a neighbor. Her quilting supplies, which had lain dormant for a decade, emerged as primary because without gardening or bird feeding, making quilts for her great-grandchildren is her new *raison d'être*.

HELPFUL PEOPLE and TRAVEL

Although these life areas might seem divergent, they are combined because travel connects us to an ever-expanding pool of people who have the potential to be helpful. This domain involves helpers on any level: friends, neighbors, family members, hospice workers—anyone involved in this individual's care on a daily basis and those who just stop by to check in. It can also include remote sources for funding, groceries, medications, and items or activities that support mind, body, or spirit.

In practical terms, this relates to transportation, finding new routes, comfort with navigating a new city and the resulting changes in independence or new dependence on family members or others. Mom, who has always been fiercely independent, is now faced with a new city. She feels unsafe venturing out on routes she hasn't memorized, and avoids busy highways. Her dependency on mass transit and friends or family has increased and therefore her sense of autonomy has suffered in ways I hadn't predicted.

Summary and Major Points

1. Each person comes to the choice of moving from a different perspective.

2. Moving "away from" is not enough. We must know what we are moving toward.

3. It's important to know what you are seeking as a result of the move:

- Lifestyle change;
- Smaller footprint;
- Family proximity;
- Creative pursuits;
- Health care;
- Improved mobility;
- Location for elderly parent;
- New challenges/business.

4. Every move/organization/project starts with knowing that something is changing or needs to change.

5. Old rules that make it difficult to know what we WANT:

- Be grateful for what you have;
- Work before pleasure;
- Don't get excited;
- Well, I know what I don't want.

6. Defining needs according to life domain or aspect:

- Health;
- Activities;
- Family;
- Finances;
- Reputation/Connections;
- Creativity/Vision of the future;
- Helpful People.

Suggested Activities

The following questions can be used for self-discovery as the helper, or done with your parent and discussed to stimulate insights and conversation about important issues and the heart's desire. As helpers, we are integral to the process, and for many life domains, there are crucial intersections between parent and adult child. Some of these activities will ask that the question be written with the dominant hand (the one used automatically when writing) and answered with the non-dominant hand. Relax and have fun with this. The left brain, typically the logical, linear side, is often the critic that tells us why we can and cannot do a thing. The right side (frequently the non-dominant) is more non-linear and creative and can give rise to ideas and approaches the left brain cannot consider. Answering with the non-dominant hand can access information in a different way and offer new insights.

1. Close the eyes and sense what life feels like being healthy, centered, and content. What colors, sounds, people, and sensations emerged?

2. Imagine days spent or work done in the new home. Using the **dominant** hand, write the question: "What would I do with my time, if I had all the money and time in the world? *Answer with the **non-dominant** hand!*

3. The realm of spirituality and wisdom includes intuition. Think about times when intuition has guided you. What gut-feelings come up about this move and how are those feelings being honored?

4. Imagine an ideal world where family and friends are there when needed. How would that be the same or different from the current situation?

5. When finances are considered, what feelings come up? What images does financial comfort bring up?

6. How would your parent like to be known or remembered by people in the family and community? What balance between private time and social interaction is optimal?

7. Are contracts with self, honored? For example, is the commitment to take more personal time being honored? With the **dominant** hand, write the question, "In what ways are agreements NOT honored? *Answer the question with the **non-dominant** hand.*

8. When you think of your future, how would you like that to look and feel? Include in this vision your connection with children and creative outlets or hobbies you might like to pursue.

9. When help is needed with a problem, emotions, or chores, is it generally available? What engenders your parent's feeling of being cared for? Insights regarding this issue can help us provide what is truly needed, instead of acting on assumptions, which may miss the mark entirely.

4

The Art of Asking Questions

To Keep or Not to Keep: That *is* the Question

Before you or your parent get too teary-eyed over the anticipation of doing without some belongings, let me share a story of my own downsizing, even though it was for a different purpose. In my young and foolish twenties, my new husband and I decided to put our "worldly goods" in storage and sail away into the sunset on a 29-foot sloop. We were hungry for adventure, had the time and no children, and had fantasized about dangling our feet in blue water, sipping Piña Coladas and watching the sunset. So we packed up, dividing things into two categories. The first consisted of articles to put into storage for setting up home when we returned to normal lives (whatever that meant). The second, much smaller category was comprised of a handful of necessities and niceties, which would fit into the VERY limited onboard storage (the equivalent of several large suitcases). Our quota included safety equipment and foul weather gear for the numerous storms that were to hit us later on.

This process meant deciding ahead of time what items were life savers (literally), what was necessary to carry for basic functions, what few belongings we simply could "not live without" and a couple of splurges, just to keep some sense of our place in the world. That meant one multipurpose saucepan, a small skillet, a little black dress that could be washed in salt water, a serious first aid kit, and a few pieces of everyday clothing. Most of the hanging locker was taken up with that foul-weather gear that we virtually lived in.

Think absolute essentials and cut that in half. And you know what? It was wonderful to wake up and know the decision of what we would use, eat, wear, or read had essentially been made for us—because there were so few choices! It was enlightening, energizing, and unburdening.

I've heard similar tales from other folks who have chosen to get back to the basics and it can be liberating beyond our wildest dreams. I recognize that doing it later in life is a different process. Still, I have a number of clients who have chosen to simplify because they wanted less to manage in order to create mental and emotional space for new opportunities and evolving relationships. When I asked my mother if there were decisions she would make differently, having now settled into her apartment, without so much as a pause she answered that all those knick-knacks she thought she couldn't live without are now the very things that get in her way. Looks like we'll be doing some more thinning out.

Even though this book addresses adult children helping parents move, I recommend sharing it with your parents. This is a shared process and reading the book or portions of it together might create the opportunity to share thoughts and feelings, or a least provide a common point of reference.

Go Forth and Conquer! But How?

There's a story about setting priorities that has circulated in different forms. A professor, hoping to make his concept more concrete, presented his students with the question of whether an assortment of rocks, pebbles, sand and water would all fit into a coffee can. At first glance the answer was "no way." And in fact, when the sand was put in first, then rocks, then water, the assortment overflowed the can. However, when the larger rocks were put in first, pebbles shaken in next, with sand following to filter and sift into the remaining spaces, and water poured in last, the concoction filled the same jar to perfection. The lesson, of course, was to take care of the big stuff (rocks) first, and allow the details (pebbles and sand) to fill in between the larger pieces—water representing the flexible items that connect and flow between the others. Water has always been a metaphor for movement and adaptability. The idea relates well not only to time and life management but the management of your stuff. Of course, a large part of moving is about "managing your stuff," determining what makes the trip and what gets left out of the coffee can. Ultimately, it's about asking the right questions: those that will get to the heart of the matter and help you decide what matters most.

Defining the Rocks

So how *do* we define what constitutes the rocks (really important stuff) versus the pebbles, sand and water? Later-in-life moves are typically into smaller spaces, so some things simply have to go. As mentioned before, most of you reading this book have some connection with depression-era thinking: everything is important—someone will need it—sometime, some-where—if you keep it long enough. Others thrived in the acquisitiveness of the "me first" and "buy everything" 80s. What a disastrous combination: buy everything, and save everything! But we are not living in a depression and thank heaven for the 1960s era, which taught us to question authori-ty. And that's exactly what we're going to do: question the previous authori-ty of the rules that may have served us well in other life stages, but now may be sabotaging us. Once these are recognized, we can answers ques-tions from a different perspective and not have the "rules" answer for us.

Self-Sabotaging Rules In A Nutshell

- Throw nothing away—it will be useful to someone;
- Whoever has the most (tools/shoes), wins;
- It was a gift: keep it;
- It was inherited: keep it;
- It's expensive: keep it;
- It's wasteful, disrespectful or sinful to throw *anything* out;
- You can't give away something for nothing.

Does It Pass the Litmus Test of Truth?

Exposing some of the underbelly of these rules often gives them less power over us, allowing us to determine if they still pass the litmus test of truth. Sometimes we are simply too enmeshed in our story to see it for what it is. It's a bit like proofreading a paper we've spent weeks writing, or a book we've just authored. It's why we hire an editor! The discussion that follows can help you edit your actions.

Throw Nothing Away—Someone Will Need It

This was true in the depression era, and might have been true when raising kids and saving hand-me-downs, but most of the items kept under this rule no longer serve us. In some cases, we are actually slaves to this stuff. Now don't laugh at this, but this rule is partly what's behind the saving of plastic bags, butter tubs, pieces of foil, 2" pieces of string, stamps peeled off envelopes, little slivers of soap and ragged, outgrown clothing. This list is endless. The fact is that most of these items represent a renewable resource. Every purchase of butter or desert topping in a plastic tub results in another storage container. Chances are, we don't still have the lids to all of those containers and three drawers of them are excessive. The same goes for plastic bags, condiment packages, paper bags, and the fifth can-opener—not to mention those notebooks from high school.

Many of our parents have saved every piece of cookware they've ever owned under the veil of guilt that erupts over throwing out an old saucepan. Years before the first move, when Mom was complaining of clutter, *I* decided it would be a great idea help her by making more room in the kitchen cupboards, the contents of which would have equipped numerous kitchens. She didn't even particularly LIKE cooking—the overflow utensils were there just in case. So, with Mom's input I filled up several boxes of extras and put them in the garage storage until she could take them to Goodwill. Some time later, my sister called and informed me that Mom had put everything back in the kitchen, complaining that I'd forced her to get rid of everything. Do not depend on your parent to "fess up" to how they are really feeling about your help. This is not a characteristic of the WWII generation and is how they came to be identified as The Silent Generation. As a rule, they are not comfortable talking about feelings, and confrontation is avoided at all costs. Mom, who is extraordinary in that respect, has learned self-reflection in her later years, but it was not part of her wiring at that time.

Another justification for keeping things is something like, "My grandson, Tommy, will need it when he goes away to college in fifteen years." Forget it, Tommy is not going to want it. He'll buy a cheap set or be given one. The same goes for nearly everything except large furniture pieces, and even then, most young people won't want to haul it around. Reserve this excuse for only the most treasured or valuable pieces and those that will FIT into the new rooms.

Whoever Has the Most (shoes, tools, books, toys) Wins

The only thing having the most of anything does for you is cause you to have a cluttered closet or a non-functioning garage. Unless Dad is a professional craftsman, how may drills can he use in the new place? Tools are expensive and if still usable, they really are among the items that can be passed on. One young couple I know had a bridal shower for bride AND groom and at the top of the groom's list were tools! A good Craftsman tool set never goes out of style. Nevertheless, take along a well-equipped basic toolbox. Even if the new place has a handyman, there is always something that needs a twist of the screwdriver and it IS a security blanket. Pictures need hanging, doorknobs tightened, etc. And how long has it been since you wore those pointy toe shoes with the funky heel and the rhinestone clips? (True, pointed-toe shoes are back in, but they're not the same as those of decades past.) If the answer is more than two years ago, pass it on. Yes, some things may come back into style, but the body changes, tastes change and unless it's investment clothing you'll want something else. Community theater groups NEED vintage clothing and your folks will probably love the idea that their things are being immortalized on stage. Also, collections that held appeal twenty years ago lose their bloom as tastes and interests change. But what do we DO with them? Besides, people keep giving us things to add to that collection! The box collection I realized I have, I am now re-gifting, one box at a time. Children who come over seem to love those boxes, and occasionally one finds a new home (the box, not the child). I've also gifted rings, earrings and pearly necklaces to friends and relatives.

Gifts You Receive Must Be Kept—and Displayed

But someone *gave* it to me! WRONG! Chances are, the person who gave Mom that awful spray-painted wooden spoon didn't know her well enough to know she'd hate it. I know you may be thinking, "If I throw this away, they'll drop by next week (even though they haven't darkened your doorway in 12 years) and know I don't have it!" If that happens, tell them aliens came down and chose it to take back to their planet, because that's about the same likelihood as this long lost relative coming to visit! Second, guilt is an overrated emotion. Reconsider if you're thinking we have to keep it to avoid hurting their feelings. Besides, moving is a great excuse for giving things away or "losing them." Sometimes there are legitimate reasons to keep something that's not our style or we don't use: your grandson made it for you. This makes your Mom's heart sing—keep this one. Keeping something as an act of respect should be reconsidered if seeing it every day triggers feelings of resentment, being discounted, burdened or overwhelmed. If you're still unsure, some of these can also be re-gifted; just be sure it's not given back to the same person. Sharing it with someone who really appreciates it is a wonderful way to honor the gift.

It's Disrespectful to Get Rid of Inherited Belongings

Wrong again, if that's the only reason they are being kept. The fact is, some people in a family become the "designated keeper" simply because *no one else will do it.* It's the game of "you're it" gone wrong. Evaluate whether an item is kept using other criteria. There is absolutely nothing "respectful" about keeping anyone's belongings boxed in the attic among spider webs. Take it out, look at it and decide what has value (emotional or monetary) to you or your parents. One friend tells the story of her mother's choice of taking only one small box with her to the nursing home. It contained the personal belongings of her great grandfather when he came to America. Mom has a similar box with her daddy's glasses, my Grandmother's hand painted Chamois used in the 1900s to apply face powder and a few silver dollars. You may need to store some things until the emotion surrounding them is less raw, and that's understandable. The problem with this is that the items are forgotten and tend to become dead weight. If you need to go through these with another family member, there are other ways to deal with items that may be of value. Those will be addressed in the chapter on Trouble Shooting.

Expensive Items Must Be Kept

(But I paid so MUCH for that...) The classic excuse is the dress or the golf clubs we paid too much for in the first place and now feel guilty about. So the argument goes a little like this: someday I'll wear that or learn to play golf (and therefore justify the expense.) Or—I love this one... in the back of your mind, keeping it amortizes the mistake over 20 years, so it becomes less expensive if we just hang onto it for a little longer! Somehow it becomes less of a mistake, because we can continue to feel guilty—sort of like doing penance. Let it go. If it was a mistake then, it's a mistake now and only takes up room. More to the point, I know that every time I look at the cursed thing, my mood drops all over again. Everyone has something like this in his or her closet or home. It has now become TOO EXPENSIVE TO KEEP. Someone else will love it and sharing it with someone who couldn't afford it feels good!

You Can't Give Away Something for Nothing

The need to receive financial remuneration for an item is a much more prominent value for depression-era individuals than for others. While this is partially related to the idea of economic well-being ("I can use that money for something else"), it's also related to the idea that "you don't get something for nothing." In this world-view, even receiving a symbolic amount of money is better than just giving something away. Therefore, auctions and garage sales seem attractive. Baby-boomers tend to look at the time cost or emotional cost associated with activities required to sell something and often would rather give it away than spend days or hours getting ready for a garage sale that will result in marginal funds. You have to really LIKE doing these sales for the work to be worth the gain, unless you have too much or really valuable stuff. Furthermore, the reality of strangers rummaging around in your history and negotiating it down to a few pennies is a poor match for the fantasy of making money from the sale.

So now we have *permission* to let go of all manner of things we thought we had to keep. But what about the things we really want to keep and no longer have room to store or display? How do we reconcile getting less for them than their perceived value or letting go of things we've felt we had to keep for someone else?

Perceived Value—Emotional and Otherwise

Much indecision or inability to release belongings that represented value in the past is anchored in the need to be *adequately* compensated for them in the present. This is obliquely related to the previous discussion of "Can't give away something for nothing," where we addressed items you really are ready to relinquish, but it takes on another dimension when talking about real treasures. The value could come from the actual cost of the items when they were purchased, or the emotional worth they represent now or in the past. It is a mistake to dismiss this by thinking it's "just about the money." *More to the point here is the deep longing that others will honor the value our lives have held.* One client tells the tale of helping her mother clear out her home, knowing that the clutter was beginning to be problematic for both her Mom's ability to function in her home and the rest of the family's ability to help her. Her mother's reluctance to relinquish these items had largely to do with her need to receive acknowledgement that her items (life) had been important.

Unless it's a rare antique, it's unlikely that value approximating the original purchase price will ever be received. So the next hurdle is to see that the value is acknowledged in some way. In this case, her mother agreed that belongings could be auctioned off, as opposed to being given to a charity. The auctioneer played a pivotal role in the story, providing emotional distance and a gentle dose of reality. In many cases, her mother was OK with receiving even ten cents for an item, just to show that someone valued it enough to pay. It's not always absolute value that matters, but the perception of value when another individual agrees to an exchange. Sometimes it is enough to know that the belongings are going to someone who will really *need or appreciate them*, which can translate into a homeless shelter as opposed to a charity where people just get it for cheap. It's a paradox, but at the shelter where people may not pay for the items, the value comes in their being truly needed.

Stuff Belonging to Grown-up Kids

Some of these things fall in the category of stuff we're keeping for the kids (Tom's *only* 35. Some day he'll marry and settle down...). I noticed with my sons who are in their mid-twenties and not so far from childhood in *my* mind that I have tended to hold on to things long after they have released them. I've kept some items—treasured books and timeless toys like wooden blocks, a LEGO® collection worth thousands and little metal cars—for *their* children. That's *my sentimentality, not theirs.* But there are many other things that lose their allure. Best to check with your grown kids or their kids before you just start throwing things out, but you may be surprised at the lack of sentimentality over items we have thought valuable to them. Yes, you might want to keep a few things they don't recognize as important NOW and will later, but for the most part, many of the "trea-sures" we've been hanging onto for *them* are really for *us*.

When our grown-up kids are in college or just starting out in apart-ments, it's nice to be able to hold on to items they "might be able to use" to start life with once they are launched. Certainly, there might be a few things—even furniture—they will want to have when they have a home or are no longer in such transitory stages of life. If you truly have the room to keep these belongings and you feel good about it, then do.

However, there comes a time when everyone has to take responsibility for their own stuff. Adult children need to make decisions. At some point, sooner rather than later (lest a pattern emerge), they should be given the opportunity to go through their stored belongings with the express purpose of making decisions about what they would like to take with them or pay to have stored.

If they don't care enough about them to pay for storage and they clearly are spending discretionary funds elsewhere for entertainment, consumer goods, etc., then the next question to ask ourselves is "why are WE storing them?" It could be that we are more invested in their belongings than they are, in which case it could be helpful to talk that out with someone. As a mother, I can attest to the power of the "empty nest" syndrome and the feelings and fears that go along with that. Among those I've felt—or heard about from clients—are:

- They don't need me anymore (but they'll come home to visit if I still have their stuff);

- I'm no longer useful (but I can be useful as the clearing house for their stuff);

- I'm helping them by storing their stuff (and it would be selfish for me to want the space).

One client kept three full closets of her daughter's clothes long after the daughter had moved on to become a successful professional in her own right. Even though my client was incapacitated by her need for functional space her own home, the act of safe-guarding her daughter's belongings continued to hold her place in the daughter's life. Some of us automatically put the needs of our children above our own, long after they are capable of taking care of themselves. If the daughter "needs" the space, we don't think twice about giving it, even if we need it for our own use.

As one who's been there and been part of this process for others, let me share with you a few thoughts to ponder:

- We are NOT usually helping our children by fixing it for them or assuming responsibility for their belongings. The sooner they deal with the real decisions and costs of hanging onto the things that no longer serve them, the happier and more responsible adults, parents and partners they will be. There is ALWAYS cost to keeping things; each individual has to decide whether the cost—be it monetary, spatial, relationship, mental focus, etc.—is worth it.

- Acting as our kids' storage facility does not gauge how much our children need us. If we have enjoyed a compatible relationship with our children in the past, they will continue to want contact with us in ways that could be far more mutually beneficial. They look to family for continuity and inspiration in ways that we may not be aware of from our present vantage point,

- The caretaking of belongings is one of the ways we establish boundaries. If our kids see us setting healthy boundaries, they will be more able to do that as well. If we are feeling "put-upon," we can do our kids a favor by not passing it on. We can give them permission to say no, by saying "No" for ourselves.

Personal Dreams

There's nothing like relocating to stir up the emotions, as memories and dreams are unearthed in the process of going through our belongings. Most often, we'd just as soon not encounter those pesky feelings. Avoidance ranks high on the list of the reasons we hang onto things. It's true of going through any of our things we've amassed over a lifetime, and nowhere is it more poignant that when we're going through memorabilia or articles we've collected while fantasizing or planning for a trip, project or a dream that has not been realized.

This became painfully obvious to me when I was helping my mother relocate from her home in Baton Rouge to Lake Charles. An avid traveler and seeker of knowledge, Mom had saved clippings from the travel sections of newspaper for years—planning places to explore and trips she wanted to take. She has traveled a lot and has realized many of her travel dreams, but we never run out of plans, do we?

She had filled file cabinets and shoeboxes with these dreams and even in her current space they were beginning to crowd out room needed for other things. At one point during this first move, we were discussing what she wanted to take to the new (smaller) house, and what she was ready to part with. Making little progress, we sat on the edge of the bed and she softly began to cry. In all the years of my young adulthood and into middle age, I'd only seem my mother cry twice. Once was the event of my father's death, and the other was the time our—once-and-only—cat jumped down from his perch on the top of the refrigerator and landed with each paw in four freshly baked pies cooling on the kitchen counter for Thanksgiving dinner! (That was our last cat. From thenceforward, we seemed to have birds, turtles and one hamster.) This time, the tears came with the realization that these dreams would never be lived. They represented lost hopes and the acknowledgement that life was slowing down. And although she professed no emotional attachment to the house in which she'd lived for forty years, certainly there was the sense of loss of living in a neighborhood that had been safe, where children were raised, and friends lived and died. After a break-in, that sense of safety was shattered and replaced by a new vulnerability.

The loss of dreams is symbolic of changes in so many areas of life, including control, access, mobility, health and a sense of the future. How do we process the dreams and collections of our lives without being overwhelmed? And how do we help another person go through a lifetime of belongings and not unconsciously discount their dreams or memories in the act of dealing with the sheer mass of the project?

How Do We Get to the Heart of the Matter?

It starts with asking questions. The preceding two chapters were the query to help you define the broader categories—the field from which more detailed information can be drawn. In this chapter, I'm preparing you for the seemingly endless barrage of questions you're going to be asking during the process of going through everything in the house. The previous chapters lay the foundation upon which all of the following decisions will be based. Only when you know the general direction of your quest (e.g., what you want in the Nine Life Domains) do you start determining the specifics of how to bring to reality the vision you're painted in your mind's eye. As you go through every closet, dresser, box of memories, cabinet after cabinet of dishware, rubber bands, paperwork, paintings, gifts from kids and grandkids, the paperweight Mom got in the Grand Canyon in 1942, there are going to be LOTS of questions you'll be *tempted* to ask, such as:

- "Hey Mom, do you really want *keep* this old thing?"

- "Do you *really* need 26 of these little cottage cheese thingies?"

- "What in the world are you keeping *this* piece of junk for?"

- "You don't really want to keep this picture of Aunt Henrietta, do you? You never liked her..."

- "Dad! You *still* have this? *No one* uses these things anymore!"

- "Oh Mom, you don't actually *wear* this, do you?"

You get the picture—and these are the polite versions. I've overheard most of them, thought ALL of them in one form or another, and asked one or two of them. Yes, I know better, but sometimes exasperation wins and the truculent teenager is given voice. I admit it, I have lapses. But every mediator will agree that asking the "right" question is not just a skill; it's an art form and we're not always conscious enough to monitor every word we say. When working with family, we are all dysfunctional in some dark corner of our lives, and terrible things can spill out of our mouths.

I can't tell you how many times I've heard tales of woe from students and clients about family rifts, and friendships torn asunder as the result of a move or organizing project gone wrong. It usually starts with a question or a statement born out of a desire to help, but spoken in frustration, judgment, fatigue or lack of consciousness. This is the way it goes...

> **Friend/Spouse:** "Why in the world are you hanging on to this old thing?
>
> **Response** "I love that memory—I wore that hat when I was five—in the school play!"
>
> **Friend:** "Oh good grief—you don't *really* still want it do you? I mean, it's all moldy!"

Response: "Yes I do—put that back! I don't need anybody else telling me what to do!"

(Soon to be) Ex-friend: "Well—I would *never* keep such a thing. I'm letting it go. It's for your own good..."

Response: "Please leave! I don't need your help and you're upsetting me."

Ex-friend: "Well, I was JUST trying to help!"

And there goes the friendship... The line-in-the-sand has been drawn and there's no turning back. One client shared the story of a rift caused from just such an interaction; it has lasted nearly a decade and reconciliation seems unlikely.

Owning the Solution

We can all ask questions, but the way we ask can make the difference between alienating someone or putting them on the defensive instead of communicating your real interest in knowing what's important to them. More than a decade ago, I embarked on what I thought might be a second career in the field of Alternative Dispute Resolution and became certified as a Mediator. As someone who loves solving problems, I thought this would be a perfect fit. Imagine my dismay when I realized the role of a mediator was NOT to offer solutions! Instead, we were taught to guide the parties to discover their own solutions. We weren't to *suggest, imply or otherwise LEAD our clients to resolution.* Well, that stung! Here I was ready to solve the problems of the world and was told NO! The goal was to create *ownership* of the solution, and that only comes when the parties themselves participate in developing the options. I decided I could live with that and proceeded forward, discovering along the way, how hard it was to keep my great ideas to myself and come up with the right questions instead!

In the process, we discovered the underlying hopes, fears and interests that drove a conflict. The "right" questions were typically open-ended in nature, as opposed to the more automatic "why" questions, which invite yes/no or either/or responses, announcing a *position*, but little more. One of the perks of using this approach is that in the time it takes to think up a question, we are saved from our baser selves who might have thrown down the gauntlet with those challenges that fly out of our mouths fully formed having never have been screened by our internal editor or good sense.

Of course, outside the professional domain of mediation or therapy with clients, one isn't held to the "don't suggest" dictum. Thank goodness, because often a suggestion might open up options it would takes hours to get to otherwise. Sometimes there's no TIME to gently extricate an idea. Just knowing when to use what question or action will save you time and grief.

Having mediated everything from "barking dog" disputes to custody battles, I've relied on what I learned a great deal with friends, family and business. It has pulled me back from the brink of some arguments that could not have been won, and given me tender insights into the workings of my teenagers' minds and hearts. It has allowed me to know my mother in ways I'd have missed if I'd engaged from my territorial animal-brain instead of consciousness. The information that percolates up offers you an opportunity to listen with your heart, and not your ego. It allows the person being questioned the chance to step away from their my-way-or-the-highway position and feel safe in the atmosphere of trust that is created. It tempers the distrust they may be experiencing from the fear that their history will be discounted or erased as years of memories and treasures are thrown out with the trash. It puts them back in the driver's seat of their lives.

Julie Tipton, one of my favorite Austin clients, volunteered this list of statements that *no one* should use in the act of helping another. Notice how closely it matches the list of questions "you'll be tempted to ask."

- "That's garbage, you need to just throw that away."
- "You're NEVER going to use that!"
- "Just *give* the stuff away."
- "That will never fit again!"
- "You don't need that!"

The bottom line is that no one likes to be managed or treated like a child, least of all our parents or spouses. We each have our own style of handling conflict and we are most likely to fall back on the style we learned in our family-of-origin, because we've had so much time to practice! Did you learn to Compete? Collaborate? Withdraw? Avoid? or Accommodate?

Perhaps you'll recognize some of these tendencies identified by The Thomas-Kilman Conflict Mode Instrument (2002):

Mode	Goal	Sounds like
Competing	To Win	"My way or the highway."
Collaborating	Win-Win	"Two heads are better than one."
Compromising	Middle Ground	"Let's Make a Deal."
Avoiding	To Delay	"Do it tomorrow."
Accommodating	To Yield	"It would be my pleasure."

Turn Disagreements into Resolution

In a class I facilitate with realtors, Turning *Conflict Into Closings*, these tools are used to help agents identify and manage the skills each party brings to a conflict. It's possible to turn disagreements and hurt feelings into positive outcome and resolution by understanding our own instinctive approach to conflict and learning how and when to use other approaches.

During relocating, opportunities for a difference of opinion and competing needs come up daily—sometimes hourly! Every mode has its appropriate use, and there is a consequence to either over-using or under-using a mode. For example, there is not always TIME to *collaborate*. When safety issues are concerned, the absolute statement of "we're doing it this way" (*competing*) may be necessary. This may be the case in this instance: "Dad, we HAVE to have handrails and a seat in the shower. I'm concerned for your safety."

When we really do need time or more information, *avoiding* can be appropriate. This opportunity came up when discussing the asking price for Mom's house. Her friend had told Mom she should be able to get at least (an exorbitant figure) for her home, because *Her* home had just sold for a similar amount. Oh boy! I *avoided* suggesting a price and offered to contact a realtor for a market assessment.

Compromising or accommodating might be best when we really do need a quick solution, the stakes aren't particularly high and meeting in the middle offers a quick fix. So when Dad wants bring every birdhouse he's every made with him to the new condo and you know there's no place for them,

Compromising or accommodating might be best when we really do need a quick solution, the stakes aren't particularly high and meeting in the middle offers a quick fix. So when Dad wants bring every birdhouse he's every made with him to the new condo and you know there's no place for them, suggest meeting half way and offering to hang a few on a wall as a happy collection. He then feels his work is appreciated and honored and you've found a graceful way around the obstacle.

No matter what the disagreement is, it's always good to know what we, ourselves, bring to the table, know when it's appropriate and when it gets in our way. If you're participating in this process for yourself, the same insights and questions can help break through your own defenses to the core feelings and attitudes. So here's a short course in...

The Art of Asking Questions

Whether sorting through belongings to determine what stays and what goes, or delving into the larger discussion of the Nine Life Domains, the general goal is gathering useful information about feelings and priorities, both of which tend to fall into a constellation of needs identified by Fisher and Ury as: "security, economic well-being, a sense of belonging, recognition, and control over one's life." From my experience with mediations and clients, I would add to that list "a perception of value or acknowledgement," which is a little like recognition, but often mixed with concepts of money and of special relevance for those who have come through the depression. In the stories that appeared throughout this chapter, you can see issues of **security** in the story about Moving Boxes; **a sense of belonging** in the story of the client who acted as caretaker for her adult daughter's clothing; **control** of one's life in the story of Personal Dreams; **recognition** in the experience of the woman who kept her newspaper articles; and both **economic well-being** and **value** in the story of items being auctioned for mere pennies. The decisions one makes are more often based on emotional underpinnings as opposed to logic or reality. Getting to those deeper issues will be easier if you understand how to use four basic types of questions: closed, leading, why and open-ended.

CLOSED QUESTIONS ("Did you want this?")

Closed questions are worded to get a "yes" or "no" answer, or very brief answer.

Positive aspects:

- Make facts more clear;
- Get a quick, brief answer.

Negative aspects:

- Stops the conversation;
- Can create hostility;
- Implies your position.

LEADING QUESTIONS ("You don't really want this, do you?")

A leading question both asks and answers the question.

- It tells the other person what YOU think;
- It tells the other person YOUR view of the RIGHT answer;
- In legal jargon it would be: "Asked and answered."

WHY QUESTIONS ("Why do you want that?")

Ask for an explanation or justification.

Positive aspects:

- *Can* sound friendly.

Negative aspects:

- Sounds like cross-examination;
- Puts someone on the spot;
- May make someone feel defensive.

OPEN ENDED QUESTIONS ("How can you see using this in the future?")

Worded to get as much information as possible.

Positive aspects:

- Asks for more information, thoughts, ideas, opinions, or feelings;
- Shows an interest in what the other person is feeling or has to say.

Negatives aspects:

- Takes more time;

- It isn't always needed.

Listening With the Heart

Our new questioning skills will help us only if we listen to the answers with our hearts as well as our minds. Listening is not just hearing; it's paying attention as much to what is not said as to what is. It is listening without always trying to "fix it," and being able to demonstrate through our responses that we are paying attention. As Jacobs and Jacobs suggest in their book *Zip Your Lips* (1999), "Just, listening without speaking is often the 'treatment of choice'." Although their book is written as a parent's guide, at the stage we are moving our parents there are times when the roles become blurred and we assume the role of the parent. Regardless, listening without fixing often requires restraint.

At all times, the ability to listen and respond with appropriate body language and expression is an important skill. It communicates to the speaker that we are fully engaged. Being able to reflect back is also useful in that it verifies that we are on the same page and that we have understood while giving the speaker the opportunity to correct any error in our understanding of either the facts or the feelings communicated.

The stories that follow show just how much information can be gleaned from the process of useful questioning and active listening. In dealing with emotional processes like moving, especially later in life, answers contain the language of facts and the language of emotions. Learning to translate both results in deeper understanding of where our parents and we are coming from. This illuminates the path ahead.

Journey into The Past

Don't be surprised if these questions take you on a journey into the past, unearthing some long buried, subconscious material. There's a lot of rich information available and the connections you make will surely help you deal with your mounds of belongings, but the real treasure is that it can change the way you move into your future. As you may have noticed, this is not just about physical stuff and the literal move; it's about the emotional sub-strata that define relationships, habits and patterns.

Little Boxes

When I was growing up, I needed more order than was in evidence in our household. I hadn't realized the insidious manner in which generalized lack of structure and emotional chaos had defined my life until I was relaying to June, a Jungian therapist I worked with for two years during my divorce, the story of my collecting little decorative boxes and being the organizer in my family.

I didn't even realize I *had* a box collection until my sister gave me a beautiful Russian treasure to add to it! "Thanks, but I don't have a collection," I said. I was shocked when I gathered up around fifteen little boxes scattered throughout the house. Separately, each holding some treasure of jewelry, keys, paper clips and such, they didn't seem like a collection. But altogether, it was a revelation! When I came across the first cedar box I got at age five when we went to the Painted Desert, I realized I'd been boxing things all my life. We finally got back to the realization that boxes were one of the ways I'd chanced upon to create order out of the chaos that was my childhood. I was the one who needed a clean house, and I was also the one who would always put treasures into categories and either mentally or literally box them up. So boxes became a metaphor for safety and cataloging memories.

Living Out of Boxes

One client I worked with came from a childhood characterized by so many moves, she had literally learned to live out of boxes and never store her belongings in chest of drawers or other forms of more permanent storage. As a little girl she'd learned she and her mother wouldn't be anywhere long enough to settle in. When it came time to move—and it always would—everything would be ready to go. I'd met her in a Clutter Busting class I taught, but her asking me for help was the result of an eviction warning. Although she'd been in her apartment for a few years, she had never unpacked most of her boxes and the landlord told her she had three days to clean up or get out.

It took some real discussion and soul searching for her to be able to part with her cardboard. Even when boxes were emptied, she insisted on storing them. Over time, she was able to let go of many of them, but only when we were able to devise a system that would allow her to move quickly if she had to. The transition from boxes to something more functional came via transparent, plastic stacking drawers on rollers. A few days after the initial cleanup, her unit flooded—and had she still been living out of boxes, everything would have been ruined. Now in a new apartment, she became terrified of being evicted again. At this point her memory of having to move out in the middle of the night had been replaced by the threat of having to move if she *didn't let go of old patterns.*

Another interesting discovery of this client was her response to a clean and orderly space. Although it was necessary for her to stay in her apartment, her first response was that it felt alien and exposed. The clutter she had lived in had become her identity and felt safe. The paradox was that this perceived "safety" became the very thing that created her vulnerability brought on by the threat of eviction. At last contact, she had settled into a significantly more comfortable relationship with living like an adult; had learned new skills in organizing and creating a living space, and was working with a therapist to resolve issues remaining from a childhood on-the-move.

Belongings as Identity Markers

It's long been recognized that our possessions are associated with our identity. Thousands of years ago, humans adorned the cave with drawings to tell stories, record events and—one can only assume—to embellish. Tribes became known by their markings, the headdresses they wore, the colors they hung from everything from shields to dancing staffs. Religious sects have identified themselves with the colors of their headdresses and vestments; teenagers with body piercing and the latest clothing fad; soccer moms with SUVs... and the list goes on.

In the military, where lack of personal identity is paramount in getting new recruits to become a cog in the wheel of a larger military machine, the first requirement is that they shave their heads and relinquish all of the clothing they arrived in. In fact, that clothing must be sent back home. I've said before that, as a Mom, it feels really creepy to get that identity shipped to you in a cardboard box!

Is it any wonder that we resist letting go of the remnants of pieces of our lives? One client carried with her every newspaper (the entire newspaper) that contained one of her articles written during her career as a freelance writer—20 years ago. They took up most of an already over-taxed garage and a good deal of interior closet space. She voiced the fear that those articles may have been the only important work of her life, and if she parted with them, she would let go of the last vestige of the talent that had created this much sought-after work. We settled on her going through the papers and keeping those that represented her best work. In this way, she was able to honor her past in a way that didn't encroach on her present. When your ties to the past begin to encroach negatively on your identity or practical needs in the present, it's time to re-evaluate. Another way to honor a talent put on hold is to recapture it in other ways and bring it into the present.

Ghosts in the Checkbook

A very well traveled and highly educated older client of mine had an issue with paying bills. This is not uncommon among folks with clutter problems and is rather a benchmark symptom for adults dealing with ADD. There's always the fear that you'll discover you've forgotten something that has resulted in negative consequences like late fees, having your account frozen, etc. It was when she asked *me* to write the checks that I began to dig a little deeper. She had no trouble keeping vast diaries of personal feelings and experiences, so I wondered what was at the root of this aversion to writing checks since she had the funds to cover them. When I asked some open-ended questions, it came out that when she was a little girl, just learning to write and form sentences, she wrote a thank you note to her grandmother. Her mother was a critical and overbearing woman, prone to verbal and physical abuse. She humiliated her, saying her writing was an embarrassment. Further, she was told NEVER to let anyone see how stupid she was.

Years later, this manifested in excruciating embarrassment and pain when she might have to write something that would be seen by someone else. Her diaries were not for public consumption and therefore not subject to the same scrutiny. She would rather pay someone significant sums of money to write her checks rather than to re-experience this humiliation.

We can all find ghosts in our childhood closets. Most families are dysfunctional in some way or another. As adults we have options we didn't have as children, and as any good therapist will tell you, things that served to protect us as children sometimes sabotage us as adults. A professional organizer can help you get a handle on your environment; a good Feng Shui consultant can help you with making sweeping life changes by working with your intentions and your physical space; and a good therapist with whom you connect can be useful in helping you resolve past issues driving current behaviors that are no longer in your best interest.

Right and Wrong

In working with yourself or a loved one, the right questions and thoughtful responses can help gently guide you through the process of deciphering the need to keep certain things and let go of others. This is a process, and there is no right or wrong to what you keep—only that it continues to support you in a meaningful way. That having been said, impasses do happen when we least expect them. Focused as we are on the best of intentions, asking all the right questions and being emotionally available, things for which we are not prepared still manage to surface, leaving us dumbfounded and out of options. What to do?

The authors of the book *Crucial Conversations* (Patterson and Grenny, 2002) offer three skills that can lead us out of the dark. Paraphrased a little they include:

- **Apologize** when appropriate. I would add to that, apologize when you can do it and feel authentic and genuine. A forced apology seldom does the trick.

- **Contrast** can work when there's just been a misunderstanding of what you meant to communicate. It includes a statement of what you DON'T mean and what you DO mean. You might say, "I would never want to hurt your feelings, and I do want to completely support you in this process."

- **Commit** to finding a common purpose by understanding what the other person really wants, then brainstorming to create strategies for achieving that purpose.

Sometimes, just stepping away and shifting the focus is all that is needed. When we can focus on the things that are working and values or purposes we share, the event that caused the impasse becomes less important. When we see old patterns emerge, or fear becomes anger, and we really do need time to cool off or get more information, simply withdrawing can give everyone time to shift. We can admit we're frustrated and suggest a break, or retreat to doing something less challenging. When working with family, ideas can be heard as mandates and when we relinquish control of the outcome, the other person is empowered to make a decision that comes from reasonableness rather than from defensiveness.

Now that you have some coping strategies under your belt, let's get to the practical aspects of how to start and how to pack. How do you take a houseful of stuff and start making sense of it so you can make well-informed decisions?

Summary and Major Points

1. Downsizing means asking questions about priorities and what stays or moves with us.

2. Self-sabotaging thoughts include:

- Throw nothing away—it will be useful to someone;
- Whoever has the most, wins;
- It was a gift—keep it;
- It's expensive—keep it;
- It's wasteful to throw anything out;
- You can't give away something for nothing.

3. Interferences to releasing things that DO matter:

- Perceived value;
- Stuff belonging to adult children;
- Personal dreams.

4. Getting to the heart of the matter requires knowing HOW to ask questions.

5. Things NOT to say or ask:

- That's garbage; you need to just throw that away;
- You're NEVER going to use that;
- Just give the stuff away;

- That will never fit again;
- You don't need that.

6. Know your conflict style and how to use others:
   - Competing;
   - Collaborating;
   - Compromising;
   - Avoiding;
   - Accommodating.

7. Knowing how to ask a question helps get to deeper issues:
   - Closed questions (yes/no);
   - Leading questions (asks/answers);
   - Why questions (demands justification);
   - Open—ended questions (seek information).

Suggested Activities

Some of the following questions can guide conversations with your parents about belongings and their value, both monetary and emotional. Others will help to identify issues that might arise as the result of growing up in different generations.

1. Are there dreams your parent(s) want to pursue or feel they will be leaving behind in the upcoming move?

2. What items represent home or identity the most?

3. What do they identify as the driving force behind keeping things (i.e., expense, guilt, identity...)?

4. What paradigm gaps do you recognize between you and your parents or those you are assisting with the move?

5. How might these differences impact your approach or interactions when moving?

5

Troubleshooting the Nine Life Domains

Now that you've given some thought to what you would like your life to look and feel like in each of the nine areas, and have been introduced to the art of how to approach the questions that will come up, let's see what specific questions might be addressed to optimize *function* in each category. The initial tier of questions dealt with desires and aspirations in the creative, emotional and intuitive (right brain) side of the equation. The following questions target *actions* that can be taken to move you closer to your goal of creating a new home that supports your parents' lives in every area of life. These questions address specific target points and can stimulate thought for other issues unique to your circumstances—issues that might be resolved with a simple fix now to avoid more dramatic actions later.

Many times, a series of obstacles develops so gradually we don't realize it until life falls apart like an old car we've neglected. It's a matter of identifying the particular item that is not working; in the car analogy, you don't condemn the whole car because the brake lights aren't working. Your parent may not need assisted living if reorganizing the space, creating a delivery system for medications, or getting a hearing aid will work. Think of the questions that follow as a trouble-shooting guide for:

- Aging in place;

- Choosing a new place for yourself; or

- Planning the move for your parents.

Planning Ahead

Planning ahead for contingencies relieves an enormous amount of stress in the process of sorting, packing, and designing life at the destination point. I am most likely to discover inadequacies in my own life when I'm really rattled, under emotional stress, sick, or in a hurry. Unfortunately, these are the least likely times to be able to problem-solve, since blood flow to the brain varies under stress and cognition takes a back seat.

Research (Center for Functional Neuroimaging, University of Pennsylvania, 2005) shows that areas of the brain associated with negative emotion are actually excited during stress, increasing negativity and vigilant behavior. Taking time with planning now will lower the crisis-quotient later. Some of the questions that follow address healthy, active lifestyles while others are phrased to generate ideas related to health concerns. All may be relevant to the stage of life in which you find yourselves at present, and serve as a guide for later issues. It's not uncommon to be processing both types of moves simultaneously, so answer those relevant to your situation!

Many of the following questions address the routine aspects of daily living, those particulars that can drive you crazy if they're not "right," and make life seamless when thought of ahead of time. In thinking about Mom, I recall talking to her about her medications: which ones she takes on a daily basis, and which are backups (antihistamines, digestive remedies, poison ivy lotion and so on). All of the non-prescription and/or backup meds were grouped in a set of stacking plastic drawers in her guest bathroom, right off the hall and across from the kitchen. That way, they didn't take up space in her primary bathroom, but were easily accessible. Medications she needed on a daily basis were placed on a small turntable in her kitchen, near the stove and the refrigerator she passes many times during the day. This location was chosen because it matched her routine at her previous home and it kept things visible. Personally, it felt like clutter to me, but I had to defer based on HER needs, not mine. Shortly after she moved in, I noticed this neat arrangement had turned to chaos with all sorts of other back-up meds littering the counter. Sometimes our best-laid plans don't work. We cannot change 80 years of habit, nor should we try.

Take mental notes on how your parent operates intuitively or habitually, and try to re-create this routine in the new place. Routine becomes more and more relevant if dementia (i.e., senility) begins to creep in, and memory of where things are placed begins to fade. Critical items have to be kept somewhat visible for them to be remembered, both in terms of schedule and locations. That being said, it doesn't mean the house needs to look like a pharmacy or smell like one. Medications can be labeled on the top of the bottle with permanent marker and put in an open, attractive basket, kept in sight to accommodate both function and aesthetics. Focusing on function alone results in constant reminders of life being reduced to maintenance, illness, or reduced capacity. That creates a mental feedback loop that worsens matters.

Use the questions that follow to help you identify needs, then find a way to keep the planned arrangement handy, visible and attractive. There are so many wonderful storage options, fabric possibilities and self-care aids. So, just because age moves in, beauty doesn't need to take a back seat. In areas such as personal hygiene, we no longer have to have a shower that looks like it came from a General Hospital to be safe and functional. There are beautiful non-skid tiles, handsome indoor-outdoor carpets that accommodate moisture, good-looking shower seats, and wonderful massaging wand, hand-held showers that make bathing easy AND support a beautiful bathroom. We no longer need to feel like a patient in our own homes.

HEALTH

The older we get, the more our energy and resources are consumed by health-related issues, even if it's just *staying* healthy and active. The more we can do to integrate activities, nutrition, medications and rituals by making them intuitive and/or accessible, the better the quality of life.

- **What activities do your parents enjoy that might help maintain a healthy lifestyle?**

- **How accessible are those activities?**

- **What needs to be done to assure that nutritional/dietary needs are met?**

- **Is health information stored for easy access by self, parent or a caregiver?**
  - Insurance;
  - Medical records;
  - Phone numbers;
  - Location of doctors' offices.

- **Are medication-needs being met? If not, what would help?**

- **Where are they most likely to FIND their medications?**

- **Are medications/supplements easy to reach and strategically located to accommodate their schedule?**

- **Can they *remember* what the medications are for?**

- **Are medications easy to open? Labels and dosages readable?**

- **Is a medication timer or organizer needed?**

- **Is clutter impacting cleanliness and creating allergies?**

  If so, what is your plan to deal with it?

- **Are there disabilities to be addressed, including:**
  - Hearing loss
  - Impaired Vision
  - Memory Loss
  - Parkinson's Disease
  - Dementia
  - Mobility
  - Memory Loss
  - Alzheimer's

- **How do they remember doctor visits? Calendar? Reminder calls?**

- **Are first aid kits, heating pads, ice packs, etc. easy to access?**

- **Would any furniture or equipment help support health or comfort?**

CAREER and ACTIVITIES

Whether we are still involved with a career or business, looking toward retirement or moving into an assisted living facility, activities keep life interesting, give us something to look forward to and help keep us vital. Even if we are down-sizing, honor some space for hobbies and pastimes. Once our time is freed up for leisure, we need room to enjoy what keeps us passionate about life and engaged with others who share our interests.

- **What are their pastimes? Is there adequate space for this activity?**

One woman I know spends hours each day doing jigsaw puzzles. Her children bought her a special table and lamps for Christmas and set them up in a seldom-used guest room.

- **What brings your parent joy and companionship?**

Whether it's bird watching, cross word puzzles, church work, other volunteer work or playing bridge, how available is it and can your parent get there? Are there others nearby with whom this interest can be shared?

- **How accessible are entertainment supplies (games, computer, reference books)?**

For example, my mother loves to do the *New York Times* crossword puzzles and has several shelves of reference books. These are kept within arm's reach of her chair in the living room, so she can watch the birds and do the puzzles at the same time. These need to be separated out first and arrangements made to keep them close at hand.

- **Are all supplies that relate to a project stored together, as much as possible?**

A little organizing can make the difference between accomplishment and disinterest.

SPIRITUALITY

Remember that spirituality is not just about religion, it's about feeling connected to a greater whole, feeling comfortable with where and who we are, feeling we are valued and feeling calm and centered.

- **What does your parent do to take care of her spiritual life?**

This could include taking more time for oneself, activities like long walks, meditating, enrolling in leisure–learning class, Tai Chi or the like.

- **How do they manage stress and emotional well-being?**

Again, a wide range of options is available and could include regular chats with a friend or counselor, exercise, deep-relaxation or meditation sessions, Yoga, etc.

- **Does your parent have a place that's really theirs in the house?**

This can especially be a problem if they live with another family. Feeling displaced causes depression, grief and a feeling of not being worthwhile. Depression weakens the immune system; so feeling you have a place that is "yours" is primary.

- **Do they belong (or want to belong) to any group that meets regularly?**

If so, is that connection honored in terms of schedule, transportation? Do you need to build in any process or schedule that makes that easier?

- **What means of transportation are available to such gatherings?**

Just knowing that a way to-and-from such gatherings is always available reduces stress in the elderly.

- **Are there members of a church or social group that can help maintain order or share errands or company?**

Local Agencies on Aging and volunteer groups often help with errands, light housekeeping and companionship.

- **Would better organization help with focus, clarity or feeling centered?**

Clutter has a debilitating effect, for most people. Reduced vision, poor mobility, and memory loss exacerbate the problem.

FAMILY

This category is not limited to biological family; it can include caregivers, neighbors, volunteers and friends.

- **What roles do biological and extended family play in this person's life?**

Are there family members nearby to help with shopping, check-ins or transportation and if so, on what basis (as needed, scheduled, emergencies only)? If so, make a list of things you/they need help with and allow helpers to choose what they would be best at. This approach usually brings in more help than if people are being assigned duties for which they are poorly matched.

- **How much time are they willing to devote to family if the move takes them closer to family and how do they fit in?**

With proximity come divergent expectations regarding visits, assistance and family gatherings. If we have not lived near family in many years it may take some time to determine availability, boundaries and schedules. Being up-front about availability and expectations can reduce hurt feelings and assumptions later.

- **Is there a current Last Will and Testament, and/or Living Will? Can you/your family find it? Have permission statements clearing physicians to discuss medical issues with specific family members been signed?**

These documents are important regardless of age, and need to be updated periodically under normal circumstances. Physicians will NOT discuss a parent's health with an adult child just because we are family, without having a signed permission statement on file.

- **Do all caretakers and family members know where essentials are located in the house?**

- **Are there pictures or items that need to be passed on to family NOW?**

Going through some of these with your parents now can strengthen your relationship, lend a feeling of control over the process while honoring your parent's contributions to your life, AND help with depression-era parents feeling that their lives are being honored.

FINANCIAL AFFAIRS

Finances cover not only literal income/support and reserve accounts to cover emergencies, but also one's perception of well-being, and the sense of being cared for. "Enough" is relative to needs and lifestyle—for some it means the ability to pay the utilities and for others it translates to having enough to travel or maintain hobbies.

- **Are there sufficient resources to cover needs?**

Who has access to accounts and in what frequency and manner? Some accounts allow a pre-specified number of checks per year without penalty.

- **Are any "checks and balances" necessary to keep peace among siblings who might disagree with how funds are managed?**

You can save grief later on by determining guidelines before dispersal becomes necessary, especially if large amounts are being spent for nursing care, in-home therapies, etc.

A guardianship can be arranged if siblings cannot agree, but this can depersonalize care and reduce control in areas relating to "quality of care."

- **Is financial information stored in an area where it can be accessed in an emergency? This includes the locations, account numbers, contact personnel for all CDs, insurance policies, and bank accounts: savings and checking.**

This is important regardless of age and health, but becomes more critical when family members must take responsibility. Moving is a perfect time to segment out essential documents.

- **Who is minding the store in terms of finances, bill paying, etc?**

If your parent is still able to do this independently, it will be made easier if a system that matches their needs and preferences is set up in an area of the house where they feel comfortable working. Setting up an automatic draft can help reduce stress if income is dependable.

- **Can they put their hands on receipts, bill paying supplies, statements?**

It may be located at the kitchen table, or by their favorite chair, but creating an accessible file system that matches THEIR categories and methods will help keep them independent.

EXTENSIONS INTO COMMUNITY or CONNECTIONS

As we mature, our community changes due to many factors, including children growing up and having lives of their own, the loss of friends and the changing status of our parents. Frequent and dramatic adjustments may cause us to question our roles, doubt our sense of self-worth, usefulness and value. When relocating into new communities, it's important to reinstate the sense of belonging as soon as possible.

- **What specific connections to the community at large are there: church, organizations, job, volunteer agencies, etc.? Will these help with creating a sense of home?**

Sometimes the most mundane activities done with a group, or for someone, can lend to a feeling of usefulness. It could be chopping vegetables for a pot-luck dinner, folding laundry, stamping envelopes or teaching someone how to play a game.

- **What areas of expertise or activities are they known for (volunteer work, knowledge in area of history, government, and school, .etc), and how can they be used in the new location?**

Teaching others how to quilt, giving lectures on local history, playing the piano, or other areas of expertise or talent lend a feeling of importance and continue to recognize one's accomplishments and wisdom.

- **Are there other difficulties that could be addressed by connecting with the outside world?**

Feeling uninvolved or useless is a significant cause of alienation for many people no longer engaged in work, family or other productive endeavors.

A retired CPA I know assists others in his retirement complex with tax questions, another organizes a book club and an accomplished artist gives painting lessons.

- **If so, what practical issues impact the ability to connect with the groups that are important to them?**

Transportation usually heads the list, but getting supplies organized, equipment, etc. can also inhibit involvement. Some simple fixes like leaving supplies on site, or getting a helper to carry them in and out can make the difference between isolation and community.

RELATIONSHIP

Relationships also change with mid-life and aging. At times, the parent becomes the child, a spouse becomes a caretaker, and our life-partners may no longer be partners, but custodians, alien creatures, burdens or jailers. Retirement of either spouse can be cause for celebration or concern, changing long established patterns and dynamics. Changes in health can require dramatically different living conditions and separate a couple that hasn't spent a night apart in fifty years.

- **How might your parents' relationship be affected by the move?**

Will they have more or less time with each other and how might this change things?

- **Are both parents alive and making the move together?**

The divergent needs of each must be addressed when setting up the space. While this may seem obvious, there are ways to accommodate an illness or changes in mobility without making the place feel like a nursing home. Whenever possible, make adjustments that are not constant reminders of declining health, by integrating them into an otherwise normal and comfortable environment. A functional shower for example doesn't have to feel institutional.

- **If so, how do their needs mesh or interfere with each other? Remember the nursery poem "Jack Spratt could eat no fat, his wife could eat no lean?"**

Translate that to keeping medications separate, mobility issues, habits, sleep patterns and so on.

- **Has the spousal relationship changed by illness, death or divorce? Each of these carries a different sense of loss, which can impact us physically and emotionally.**

Would grief counseling or medical attention support the process?

- **If our parents are separated from each other, how will that impact life for them and their families?**

Does the more mobile partner have transportation or telephone access to the other one?

CREATIVITY and VISION OF THE FUTURE

We might be shifting gears in response to kids having gone to college, wanting to streamline our lifestyle, accommodating a change in marital status, moving into a retirement community or moving to assisted living. Giving serious thought to what we want the next five years to look like will dramatically impact the way life unfolds. This gives the chance to more actively choose our lifestyle regardless of circumstances. Considering choices ahead of time makes even the most difficult move more bearable and successful at our destination. This is true even if those choices are limited to handwork, reading materials, access to loved-ones, and what we bring with us. Make this move count. This can overlap with the Activities domain, but is another way to think about creative juices. Not all the activities available to us are creative and it is known that humans need to have an outlet for creative energy.

- **What makes their heart sing when looking forward?**

Are there classes to take, second careers to build, businesses to grow, countries to be explored, grandbabies to bounce? A very real possibility for those confined to a more stationary existence is to write or record family history or memories from childhood. With our expanded mobility and generations living apart, the kind of history-sharing that used to take place around the dinner table or holidays spent together has all but gone. Here is an opportunity to record it for future generations.

- **What living arrangement would make those dreams more possible?**

Living in a structured community? A guesthouse behind the kids' home? A smaller home with a nod toward ease of care? A home that will welcome extended family and grandkids for the summer? The second half of life can offer both immense freedoms and the reality of slowing down in some arenas.

- **Are your parents looking at a nursing home or extended care in the near future**?

If so, how does this impact the need and schedule for downsizing?

HELPFUL PEOPLE and TRAVEL

Travel, in addition to being for enjoyment and education, might also be a large part of later life simply because our families have spread out. Not only do we meet people who might become friends and helpers, we sometimes need assistance to allow us to travel, in addition to simply receiving help from "the universe." Caregivers, while addressed under health as well, also fall into this category.

- **What kind of travel, if any, have your parents looked forward to?** Europe, to visit family, Elderhostel trips or across town to visit friends or essential errands. Not everyone wants to travel, but if it is a priority, think about their needs and what type of help, if any, will be needed to accommodate *special* needs. These might include:
  - A companion;
  - Transportation to and from the airport;
  - Pet sitters;
  - House sitters;
  - Assistance at the airport;
  - Take-along snacks, contact phone numbers, emergency care information.

- **Is there a directory of *helpful people* with contact numbers, schedules and e-mail addresses posted near each telephone? Also include:**
  - Hospice when appropriate;
  - Lawn care specialist;
  - Handyman;
  - Friends;
  - Volunteers who bring meals, do daily call-ins, etc.

- **How can neighbors or friends who routinely help be rewarded?** You might get a neighbor to check in on Mom or Dad daily or weekly and say thank you with dinners, gift certificates or an occasional handwritten note.

Summary and Major Points

This chapter presented a level of detail that provides a type of filter for making decisions about belongings: those that make the trip and those that need to be anticipated at the other end. Generally, making such a move for our parents is the result of some change in their ability to fully care for themselves in their current residence. When we are responding to such changes, the natural tendency is to focus on the immediate needs, not the more mundane day-to-day activities that sustain life beyond the crisis. This short-sightedness gets us through the crisis, but does little to help us prepare a place that meets their needs when moving into the future. The goal, of course, is thriving, not just surviving.

DOMAIN	CONCEPT	FUNCTIONAL MATTERS
HEALTH	Physical mental, emotional balance. Medical concerns. Staying healthy and active, Hearing, vision, mobility, dexterity.	Location of medications, legible prescriptions, ability to open containers, physical arrangement of space, self-care.
CAREER & ACTIVITIES	What keeps life interesting and vital: career, hobbies, volunteering, opportunities.	Hobbies, proximity of activities, transportation to and from, room to do them.
WISDOM & SPIRITUALITY	Feeling connected to life, feeling calm, centered, grounded, valued, needed. Could include religious life.	Space of one's own, privacy, access to church if desired, making a contribution.
FAMILY	Biological family, social community that offers family-like support, sense of community.	Philosophical match with the community, like minded others, keeping in touch with friends and family from before the move.

DOMAIN	CONCEPT	FUNCTIONAL MATTERS
FINANCIAL AFFAIRS	Monetary resources, feelings or reality of enough to care for our needs and desires.	Actual availability of funds, access to funds, insurance, documents and their location, Power of Attorney, day-to-day management of finances.
EXTENSIONS INTO COMMUNITY	Literal connections with the outside world, maintaining a sense of identity and expertise, integrity and authority.	Possibilities to share expertise, continue to be recognized for contributions, opportunities to teach, share and mentor.
RELATIONSHIP	Relationship with life partner or with one's "self."	Continuity of marriage or family relationship: living apart. Spousal visits. Feeling good about self.
CREATIVITY & FUTURE	Vision of the future, opportunities to express talents, be creative, express ourselves in unique ways.	Projects (quilting, cooking, music, dance), access to materials, space to do what we love, funds and access to materials.
HELPFUL PEOPLE & TRAVEL	Literally, travel for fun and receiving help from others when needed.	Proximity to airports, doctors' offices, shopping and those people who support life in other ways.

Suggested Activities

1. What are the three most important health factors your parents want to change, maintain or impact with this move?

2. Ask your parents about activities they look forward to when they get to their new home and list those below. What can you do to make them happen?

3. Which rituals or practices help them stay centered and deal with stress, and how can you help integrate this into their new life?

4. Discover and list three fun way your folks can be incorporated into family time or create new friendships in their new community?

5. What are the two most important financial factors involved with your parents' new life and how can those be positively impacted or managed?

6. List three ways your parents might like to share their talents or expertise with new friends or community? What kind of help is needed to fulfill this goal?

7. What are two things that might help support any changes in your parents' relationship if circumstances have changed their living arrangement?

8. List three ways you will set up your parents' new place to encourage their specific creative outlets, whether it be cooking, gardening, sewing, writing or helping others?

9. How will their need to travel or receive help with travel be impacted by the move and what steps can you take to see that their needs in this area are met?

6

Attracting the Experience You Want

Moving house, for yourself or another, is rife with opportunities for stress, conflict, resistance and blame. It is simultaneously abundant in opportunities to enrich relationships by being helpful; offering unconditional love and support; being compassionate, and sharing memories and laughter. We can often re-frame our history and handcraft a future that we choose instead of one that evolves via default. The character of the move we experience is largely dependent on the attitude we as helpers, facilitators, or caretakers bring to the process and demonstrate in every breath. Any major relocation is naturally filled with concern over what's ahead, and the what-ifs of life, possibly guilt, grief, joy and excitement. For our parents, this represents The Move of a Lifetime, and it is often the only move they will experience as adults after the first move away from their own parents. Moving our parents is complicated by the realization (ours and theirs) that their move represents life in its closing chapters.

> How we experience a move is so much more than the function of logistics and the obvious details. At every juncture in life, we have the opportunity to make decisions and choices about how we think, feel, respond and interact with others. Ideally, these choices are the external indicators of our intentions and internal aspirations.

When working with our families, we often experience a mixture of emotions and intentions that conflict with each other, and those conflicting emotions drive our actions. We have helped our parents make conscious choices about what they and we want life to feel like in the Nine Domains. Similarly, we can make decisions and choices about how we participate in and guide the process of helping our parents. We do this by being more aware, acting from the heart of compassion and consciously managing our thoughts to guide our emotions in the direction that matches our inner- most desires. The guidelines we apply to moving our parents can also guide us as we think of *our own roles* in each of the life areas. The insights and compassion brought to bear with family have a good home in the fertile ground of our own psyches. When we are able honor our contracts with ourselves, respond to our own inadequacies with compassion and become clear about our intentions, we are more likely to be able to externalize those characteristics when challenged by others. The circle is complete.

Demons—Fear Them or Slay Them

The crucible of working with families reinvigorates the fire-breathing demons of childhood if there are any, and we are presented with another opportunity to feed them or slay them. Two stories come to mind. When my firstborn was in the throes of his terrible-twos and just being his own mer- ry yet defiant self, I found myself screaming at him like a woman pos- sessed. For a moment, I saw the spectacle from outside myself and remember having the feeling that I was witnessing it as an observer seeing an out-of-control parent, driven by a past that now repeated itself in the demand for obedience. Horrified by the possibility that I would foist this pattern onto my own precious children, I began a systematic process of un- raveling a past that would drive our future if I didn't act otherwise. I be- came a very different parent as a result, and while I may have repeated other patterns, the unrelenting expectation of perfection at all costs was not one of them. I share this story as an example of how old patterns of the treatment we received in our families can easily be triggered. When roles reverse, it's not uncommon to see ourselves exhibiting the same parenting style we *experienced* as children. These patterns can blindside us because they may only surface in the context of our family or origin.

The second story relates to a client (we'll call her Stella) who was called to the aid of her 84-year-old Russian immigrant mother, who as a child had endured four years in a labor camp. After a lifetime of emotionally ab- using her children, the mother called the one remaining child who had tried to maintain contact. The others, two sons and another daughter, re- mained estranged and lived lives of quiet desperation: one an alcoholic, another a drug addict, one a family man torn between gentleness and mean-spiritedness. The only evidence of any tenderness in the old woman came in the form of a community of feral cats she fed from the back porch, and one she allowed to live inside as a pet. Made a ward of the state at the age of fifteen because of physical and emotional abuse, Stella was ultimately raised by an aunt. Months before her high school graduation, Stella joined the military to avoid having to live on the streets. She went on to graduate, got an engineering degree, worked as a risk-management engineer and later as an award-winning graphic designer.

Wife, mother, newspaper publisher, artist, and all around overachiever, Stella remains chronically plagued by feelings of unworthiness. Nevertheless, she was able to keep the wolves at bay until, at the age of forty-seven, she re-entered the nightmare of her mother's home. Age had done nothing to mellow her mother—the verbal abuse started immediately, as though the mother had simply been holding her breath for the intervening decades. The full flood of emotions was unleashed when Stella began packing up the little figurines her mother wanted protected in case "thieves break in (to her home) while I am in-hospital." Paranoid about people stealing from her, she berated her daughter into packing up the very items that had surrounded Stella during her years of abuse and torment. Already unhinged by the memories represented by little figurines and knick-knacks, Stella discovered an abandoned and dying kitten under the steps. Inconsolable until she was able to buy formula and a medicine dropper to nurture and love this kitten, she reasoned, "this kitten may die, but it will do so in loving arms."

In such ways, we are both driven by and given opportunity to face and at least partially salve the wounds of our past. As of this writing, Stella has returned several times to her mother's home and has learned to set boundaries and move beyond the emotional scars of her nine-year-old psyche. The result has been an improved relationship and a few rare words of praise she has waited decades to hear. Like the legendary Lotus buried in layers of mud, this relationship had lain dormant and has finally begun to bloom. Stella was able to see through her own pain and her mother's tragic past to heal a relationship she'd given up on. This healing has begun to extend other areas of Stella's life and empower her to make life-changing decisions. This is the power such moves have over our lives.

Re-Scripting Our Histories

We don't all have such tormented histories, but each of us will face some remnant of an unresolved story, that, like a thorn, works its way up to the surface. As adults we have new skills, maturity, options and support systems to re-script our histories. Some of it may require professional guidance, but all can be assisted to a greater or lesser degree by the information and techniques that follow.

> Now, more than any other time in our history, research repeatedly confirms what we've known intuitively for thousands of years: that our thoughts and emotions influence those around us.

All of us have heard tales of healing, precognition, and mental communications. Many of us have personally experienced such events. I grew up hearing stories of my great grandmother's healing work in a small town in Louisiana. My great aunt, Ivy, continued it after her mother died. Both my father's mother and her sister had many clairvoyant experiences—knowing an event had occurred before the news arrived. Many of us have had such experiences with friends or family, and in general people are more open about discussing what has come to be called the "sixth sense."

For most of my lifetime, most people have dismissed these occurrences as coincidence. Fortunately, science has finally evolved to the point that these events are not only being examined and confirmed, but partially explained. The shelves at libraries and bookstores are heavy with books about the power of thought to influence our lives, the first of which was Norman Vincent Peale's book, *The Power of Positive Thinking* (1952). Although precognition, clairvoyance, etc. may seem like a different process from positive thinking, they are related phenomena. Each has to do with the power of the mind and our ability to both send and receive information mentally and energetically. Recent research adds further dimensions to this realm of influence; thought and emotions influence not only people, pets and plants but the behavior of random event generators, photons and sub-atomic particles in general.

At the core of these realizations are findings that originated with the research in Quantum Physics and string theory. As Brian Green states so straightforwardly in his book *The Elegant Universe* (1999), we are now realizing "that everything at its most microscopic level consists as vibrating strands." In fact, particles are not particles at all, just "reflections of the various ways in which a string can vibrate." Further, these vibrating strands are in constant communication, electrons communicating by "shooting" photons back and forth at each other, whereby the photon is actually acting as a "messenger particle." This fact of communication, the depth of influence this generates, and the supporting research is the subject of many recent books, but certainly one of the most readable is Lynn McTaggart's *The Field* (2002), summarizing and translating this research into language the rest of us can assimilate. Although it is outside the scope of this book to review this research, a few discoveries have exciting relevance for the business of moving, shifting gears and all the emotional challenges these entail:

- Through the process of thought, we have the ability to synchronize our brainwaves with one another and the most "ordered" brain pattern prevails (allowing us to give calm support to those with whom we wish to connect);

- We have the ability to "shield" ourselves from intrusive emotions or intentions from others (empowering us to consciously distance ourselves from destructive attitudes of others);

- Sending another "good thoughts" for healing or calming has the same impact as if they had that thought for themselves (making it possible for us to support loved ones at a distance);

- The release of a thought or intention and its receipt by the "target" is instantaneous (enabling us to communicate our support simply by releasing the intention).

So, we have a lot of potential to impact the well-being of another person, and for that matter of ourselves. Consciously managing our thoughts and intentions presents us with a grand opportunity to be aware of our emotions, and to promote a positive outcome. Stefan Schmidt, Ph. D. of the University of Freiburg, Germany discusses how "health care professionals can create an optimal healing environment (OHE), with a special focus on which inner state and way of being in the world can create a healing intention." We have the potential to calm, support, and facilitate healing by calming our own minds and holding the intention for well-being.

While conversation can help, it is neither possible nor desirable to be in dialog all of the time. Sometimes we just ache for a way to help, to communicate or to soothe without saying a word. What a wonderful realization that we can do precisely that—by holding the desire as a thought, a prayer, or a visualization of the emotion of compassion regardless of time, place or other constraints present in very complex relationships.

Another Channel

A few years ago, one of my sons was going through a particularly tough time, having relocated to another state, knowing no one, grieving the loss of a love and dealing with weather-related blues. We had just said good-bye after a difficult conversation. He was bent on returning home. Such a move would have been a step backward for him and would have re-connected him to a social group he'd had the good sense to leave behind. Knowing my own ambivalence in the situation, I first had to become clear about the mixed message I might be sending. Finally I sat and wrote him a long e-mail, with a number of very specific reasons for staying there and experiencing some success before he made any drastic decisions. I sent the e-mail late that evening along with my love and spiritual support. The next morning he called, in a much-improved state of mind, laughing actually, and explaining why he needed to stay until he had some successes. His reasons matched those I had detailed, almost verbatim. Toward the end of the conversation, I asked if he had received my e-mail. "No," he replied, "I forgot to tell you I have a new e-mail address, but you can resend it." There was no need—he'd already received it via another channel!

Every Thought Has a Receiver

In his book, *Dogs Who Know When Their Owners are Coming Home*, Rupert Sheldrake (2000), investigated the realty behind the stories he kept hearing about pets that demonstrated their awareness that their owner was headed home. I don't know about my cat, but I remember that I usually knew when my husband was about to arrive because I heard the car door slam and the back door open moments before he actually headed down the hill. Sheldrake describes his research whereby pets and their owners were separated (sometimes by great distances) and simultaneously filmed via remote camera while pets remained in their familiar homes and owners were stationed at research stations elsewhere. Owners were instructed to mentally set the intention about coming home, at some point in time known and noted only by the themselves, not the researcher. The surprising results showed that pets responded with anticipation the *instant the intention was released*, not at the hour the owner specified for arriving.

This and other research has me fond of saying "Every thought has a receiver." Research studying "the sense of being stared at," conducted both by Sheldrake and others, shows a statistically positive correlation between being stared at and being able to sense both when it is happening and when it is not.

The point is that we communicate our intentions in ways that extend beyond the ordinary and our intentions have the ability to impact the outcome of events and our relationships. Nowhere will you experience as much opportunity (and necessity) to understand what you bring to the game as when you work with your parents and siblings. It brings to mind the poem *"If"* by Rudyard Kipling: *"If you can keep your head when all about you are losing theirs and blaming it on you, yours is the Earth and everything that's in it..."* You will find ample opportunity to test this!

I've been told of a Native American expression that one's dreams are carried to heaven on the wings of an eagle. In the realm of co-creating your reality, I would say "Our dreams are carried into manifestation on the wings of our emotions." It is not so much the thought as the emotion supporting that thought that does the attracting or influencing. Add to this the knowledge that we have more control over our thoughts and emotions than we may have understood while growing up, and we begin to actualize a great deal of control over how our dreams, aspirations and goals come into fruition.

Daniel Amen, M.D., in his groundbreaking book *Change you Brain, Change Your Life* (1998), devotes a chapter to the way thought patterns impact our brain chemistry, behavior, moods and success or failure. In the chapter on Enhancing Positive Thought Patterns, he makes this statement:

> "Thoughts have actual physical properties. They are real. They have significant effect over every cell in your body. When your mind is burdened with many negative thoughts, it affects your deep limbic system and causes deep limbic problems (irritability, moodiness, depression, etc.) Teaching yourself to control and di-

rect your thoughts in a positive way is one of the most effective ways to feel better."

What's so delicious about that is this: If our feelings contribute to our ability to influence others as the research indicates, and we can shift those feelings through the practice of thought reframing and other techniques, then we have an enormous capability to positively impact the way we feel, and influence our relationships.

Killing the ANTs

Dr. Amen has a prescribed method for changing these thoughts and the resulting emotions that he calls "Killing the ANTs" (Automatic Negative Thoughts). There are other avenues to this awareness and one of those is the spiritual concept know as the Law of Attraction, popularized by the work put forth by Ester and Jerry Hicks in their book, *Ask and It is Given* (2004). These two approaches, while radically different in their origin, both point to the same place and use similar tools. Let's look first at the information made available from neuroscience and Dr. Amen's research.

1. Automatic thoughts (the type we develop over a lifetime of repeated interactions and exposure) create synaptic pairings in the brain (a fixed neural pairing across a synapse).

2. When you have a thought, it releases a rush of chemicals in the brain and that chemical-bath results in feelings that are either positive or negative.

3. An electrical impulse results and you become aware of the thought.

4. Our emotions and the way we feel about life and events can be changed through a process called "thought reframing," which can literally eliminate the automatic synaptic pairing, form new neural associations and result in different chemicals being released. That in turn results in different feelings.

I've been teaching this concept and using the process for years with my clients, family and myself. I can attest to its working. It's an elegantly simple process, but in order for it to work one must become exquisitely aware of thoughts and emotions, the moment they occur. It requires consciousness, persistence and a shift in the old paradigm that we simply respond to the world around us as best we can. Joe Dispenza's recently published, *Evolve Your Brain (2007)* gives an excellent explanation of the neuroscience behind this process.

The concepts found in both the Amen research and the Hicks material have been alluded to in many different forms throughout history. Peale's previously mentioned work first hit the bookshelves in 1952, selling 20 million copies in 44 different languages. A more complete listing of other publications on the subject can be found at the end of this book.

A real-life look at thoughts that will make this process of moving Mom and Dad more difficult might help:

- Every move I've made has been a disaster;

- Moving Dad is going to be a pain. He knows just how to push my buttons;

- I've never had any help with moving;

- I'm just a packrat. I can't do anything about that;

- Mom's not going to like this;

- This is going to take forever.

By re-framing the above thoughts we can contribute to a more positive, soul affirming process. The re-framed thoughts might look like:

- This move could be different—I have new resources;

- Dad and I might get along fine. I know how to set my boundaries now;

- The ideas in this book will make the move easier;

- I have new ways of determining what I can let go—I'm really ready to simplify;

- I don't know that—Mom might like this;

- I don't know how long it will take—I have more experience now.

It is so easy, almost automatic, to revert to old patterns that were set up in childhood. Only those with whom we have shared deep history and extreme emotions (love, fear, hope, despair, joy, sadness) have the ability to elicit from us emotions that come right out of childhood and adolescence.

Who else besides your parent can turn you into a belligerent teenager in one breath and fill you with tenderness and regret in the next?

Changing the Dance Step

There are real challenges to moving anyone, ourselves included. It's well known that our best hope in impacting a situation is not in changing the other person, but in shifting our own responses to their behaviors. We must take responsibility for what we bring to a situation, relationship, argument or dilemma. Each of us comes with attitudes, baggage, expectations, tendencies, wounds, fears, joys and every other possible emotion. Over time, the manner in which these variables articulate with others in the transaction can form a pattern like a dance. In long-established relationships like those with family and spouses, these dance steps can be anticipated so well that before we have even completed one step, our partner is preparing to respond. Old patterns become entrenched and cannot be broken until one of us decides to change the steps. When we do that, the other person may be thrown off for a moment and try to maneuver us back into the pattern. But what happens if we don't repeat the old step? Ultimately our dance partner has two options: leave the dance floor or find a new dance step. Changing the dance step is in some ways an external method of breaking the synaptic pairing. If we do it often enough, the automatic response falls away and a new pattern or dance step replaces it.

This opportunity came up for a client who had responded to a pattern with her mother for as long as she could remember. She and her mother had fought bitterly during her adolescence, and over the years my client had learned to avoid engagement in most situations. Since they have always lived at least a day's drive away from each other, face-to-face encounters were rare and each tried to be on best behavior. If they disagreed on something innocuous and my client voiced a different opinion, her mother would snap back, "You've always had a hair-trigger temper!" Because my client seldom, if ever, lost her temper, her mother's statement got to her. As you've probably guessed, she stepped right into the snare by answering, "I do not!" And that's all it took to start the dance... But one time, she managed to consciously step back, not engage, and simply changed the topic of discussion. Her mother tried again, no engagement... It was tried once or twice after that, but it's been ten years since that incident and the pattern has never been repeated. Although it's not always that easy, sometimes it is—the shift is worth the wait and persistence.

Everyone I know has a story about visiting Mom and Dad in the family home and being horrified as they watched themselves turn back into the children they had been decades ago. The stresses of moving, loss of territory and sense of our place in the world have a cumulative impact on calling forth old patterns of defending and challenging. Even with the best of intentions, the requirement to make many stressful decisions at once can overload even the most highly trained individual. None of us are totally immune to meltdown when it comes to dealing with our folks, much as we love them.

In terms of creating the experience we want, as opposed to responding to one that we just stumble into, the key is to ask this question at every possible juncture:

"Is my emotion consistent with the outcome I desire?"

Basically, it works like this: if your intention is really to support your parent and have a good experience doing it, but you are feeling angry, resentful, anxious or fearful, then your emotion is NOT consistent with attracting a positive outcome. With these emotions in the driver's seat, you will create experiences and encounters that produce more anger, fear, and anxiety. Conversely, quantum shifts are possible if at each opportunity for conflict, you can take a breath and remind yourself of your intention and shift to a more useful thought or emotion. The most powerful of these emotions in terms of their positive influence are love, joy, gratitude and compassion. Knowing from personal experience that these are not always at the ready when you're making your umpteenth call to the telephone company and reach yet another twenty minute progression through robotic menu options, I share how this has worked for me and other clients:

- **Love** is easy to come by when we are feeling safe and compassionate, and can allow our vulnerability. In trying times, our hearts are not always as open and available, since we protect ourselves with anger and defensiveness. Sometimes, in an effort to deflect hurt, we conceal our hearts with hostile emotions. If love does not feel genuine in the moment, we might at least feel real *affection* for the personality we remember, not the one before us. It might be more realistic at times simply to appreciate the experience of the moment as one that offers contrast to what you'd really like to create.

Negative experience has its place in the scheme of things. It offers us the contrast to fully appreciate other times and think about what we DO want. One cannot appreciate the light, having experienced no darkness. One of the best resources I've had the privilege of discovering as a way to develop the heart of love and compassion is the deeply moving, yet practical *Awakening the Buddha Within* (1997), by Lama Surya Das. Subtitled *Tibetan Wisdom for the Western World,* it offers insights that ordinary men and women dealing with real life trials can embrace and internalize. Whether you are working with an aging parent and a difficult situation, or just wanting to deepen your resolve to live a life of wisdom and compassion, it offers real jewels.

- **Joy** is sometimes the most elusive sensation in that often it is not recognized until it has passed. Embrace the moments of sharing, and the opportunity to know another's innermost thoughts and emotions. There is tenderness and a gift in being allowed to witness someone's vulnerability and in that moment we can be joyful that another trusted us enough to share it.

- **Gratitude** is possible even when the other emotions may fail us. In the Buddhist tradition, there is always the invitation to discover the gift in a crisis. The full understanding of that gift may elude us for years, but with eyes to see, it is always there. Gratitude can encompass the opportunity to be of genuine service, during which we encounter second chances. Some sources proclaim that the Chinese word for "crisis" is a combination of "danger" and "opportunity." There is some disagreement on the literal translation, but the philosophy is useful. If all else fails, embrace the opportunity you have for growth.

- **Compassion** has been defined as deep awareness of the suffering of another, with or without the accompanying need to resolve it. It means seeing their situation through their eyes, without judgment; empathizing with them. Often, the anger and impatience we experience with our parents are the result of their being infinitely frustrated with their inability to hear correctly and contribute in the way they always have. I have heard from my own mother and more than a few clients, "I've outlived my usefulness." What must that feel like? Compassion doesn't mean we have to fix it, it just means we care.

With all our good intentions and sometimes because of them, we will stumble, say the wrong thing, give "the look," and lose patience. Not engaging may be the option of choice. It gives us time to shift our emotions, change the dance step, reframe our thoughts, engage in some self-care and allow the person you are assisting to do the same.

Here's an illustration of that in practice. You have spent all day going through belongings and making decisions about what gets kept and what falls away. You come across the umpteenth version of a *mathom* (a Hobbit term for an item for which no use can be found) and your Dad says he MUST have it. If you engage, out of habit, you might just trigger the line-in-the-sand to meet the challenge. It's the *principle* of the thing, you say: you've GOT to get rid of something. By not engaging you do two things:

- **First,** you will have given him the freedom to decide without having to defend his position, so you've given him back some power. This is important, because he is already feeling a bit powerless. This option allows him to decide, "not to take it" later, which is usually within a moment or two;

- **Second**, you will have demonstrated and created trust: the trust that he can make his own decisions without being coaxed or managed AND the trust that he won't be forced into a decision he is not ready to make. The next time an issue arises, he is much more likely to enter consensus and be open to suggestion. There's no line-in-the-sand.

Trust and Boundaries

I recently worked with a lovely couple in their seventies to create some order out of the chaos that had become their home. Both highly intelligent and creative souls, they had many interests and the husband was an information and detail junkie by training. As a researcher and author of many engineering textbooks, he had generalized his need to keep documents to include nearly everything else that came through his hands. There were journals going back twenty years and every catalog that came through for the past five years had been kept. We'd made quite a bit of progress the previous session with filing and Mr. Jones (name changed for privacy) left his wife and me to work alone. His leaving us was a great vote of confidence and indicated that he trusted us not to get rid of something of value.

When he left, Mrs. Jones and I felt it was clear we would be working in the office and making some decisions about magazines. We grouped categories together, ordered them by type and date and she eliminated duplicate catalogues and those that were more than two years old. All technical journals were kept and we were delighted with the progress. We had taken great care to avoid violating any of what we felt would be his guidelines. When he returned, he was terrified and infuriated that we might have thrown out something of great value because it didn't look the same. We clearly had misunderstood the signals and to this day we have not totally regained his trust *even though he has been able to find things more easily, work more efficiently and likes the ways his office functions.*

Because of these mixed signals, trust was eroded and the opportunity to do future work was delayed. His need to control was based on fear. When that is present, boundaries need to be carefully and respectfully identified. Without identifying them, they can't be honored, because we don't know where they are. Sometimes we can help to identify the nature of the fear and then work in a way that supports the underlying need. Much of the resistance to change is related to their losing independence, control of their belongings and affairs, and the knowledge that some things are slipping away. Learning new patterns, habits and locations is harder with age, so any changes need to be intuitive and honor habitual patterns where possible.

Another client exhibited advanced Parkinson's Disease and was beginning the use a small automated scooter to get around in her home. In addition to hoarding shoes and papers, she had several large and protective dogs in her home and raised pullets (baby chicks) in her kitchen! Years of purchasing different shoes that she thought would aid in her mobility resulted in her owning closets full of un-worn and now useless pairs. I helped her make decisions and whittle her collection down to only those that worked for her. Although she had helped set the guidelines for keeping or disposing of her shoes, she did become hostile and resistant periodically. My role was to step back and allow her room to mentally and emotionally process. Sometimes this meant working in another area while she sat with her decisions. Giving her that freedom and latitude empowered her to let go of far more. In doing so, she owned the decision. It's important to note that this ownership also reduces the potential for blame down the road when they are feeling powerless.

Creating the Vision

In Chapter 3 I mentioned that it's not enough to know what we are moving "away from." We need to consider what we're moving toward as a way of ensuring that we create what we really want at our destination. Otherwise, we may find ourselves with the same issues, just at a different geography. It's the difference between the sadness of "away from" and the anticipation of "toward" that I'd like to talk about in this chapter. That difference impacts day-to-day mood, decisions, and even how quickly the house sells after the move. Admittedly, there are times when health, safety or financial requirements leave us few options, and it is harder to generate interest in the next stage, which may be a convalescent home or Alzheimer's facility. Still, unless the person moving is medically unconscious, there are still options to consider: what pictures to take, an afghan for the bed, mementoes, the color of the walls or the drapes—the small things can make a big difference. Even if we are wrapped in the excitement of the moving *toward* mindset, it's seldom as clear-cut as one-or-the-other. There are mixed feelings regardless.

I've worked with many real estate professionals and bought and sold quite a few places myself, both as a homeowner and as an investor. One factor in the Real Estate industry is whether the seller is really happy about the move and is looking forward to the next stage. Homes that are on the market due to divorce, illness, financial disruption or any other kind of loss tend to move slower. They stay on the market for a longer period of time. Experienced agents have a long litany of experiences where properties stayed on the market for longer than they should have given their price and condition, because prospective *buyers* sensed something uncomfortable about the property. Folks couldn't usually verbalize it—it was just a feeling, but it is consistent across the market. In each of those cases, the sellers shared a feeling of moving *away from* that is characterized by grief, fear, resentment, uncertainty and loss. Sellers who are happier about the move, even though any move can be stressful, are more likely to be filled with a sense of adventure—excitement and anticipation over making the new place home, decorating it, exploring community and discovering themselves in a new way. This excitement permeates everything about the move. In some the excitement is spontaneous; in others it can be generated with a little coaxing and creative visualization.

One approach is to get the floor plan out and talk about colors, where furniture will go, where things will be placed, and how your parents will make it theirs. If there is a yard where planting can be done, it really helps to bring cuttings or plants from their old yard to the new one. If there is no yard, some plants can be potted for inside or the balcony or patio. The grief over leaving plants that may have come from dear friends can be lessened by giving them to others to plant in their yard. Again, knowing that some- one else is appreciating or taking care of things we love helps us move for- ward. This is also a great opportunity to change color schemes and use furniture in a different way to make it feel as though you've completely re- decorated. Lists of places to visit, day-trips, hobbies and discoveries can be made so that little time is lost on the other end in finding out more about the place.

Another way to create excitement is to use the process of *visioning* men- tioned in Chapter Two. Described in depth in a book by the same name, *Vi- sioning: Ten Steps to Creating the Life of Your Dreams* (2000), Lucia Capa- cchione takes the reader on a journey into the process. For those who would like to experiment, here are the basic steps used by many creativity and intuition coaches. A process I've used with clients goes like this:

Get together the following materials:

- Magazines (any topics that interest you);

- Fabrics if you have some you've been lusting after;

- Color samples you're thinking about (remember Mom's peach and greens);

- Poster board, scissors, glue-sticks;

- Several kinds of music for background (nothing that will take you backward emotionally);

- A couple of hours of uninterrupted time.

Phase One: Put on some fun music, happy music that makes you want to move your body!

- Set a timer for 30 to 45 minutes.

- For the next 30 minutes or so, tear pictures that "grab" you! Don't analyze or trim; just tear them out without mentally editing them or trying to figure out why you like them.

Phase Two: When your timer goes off, choose some different music and start the next phase:

- Cull through the pictures and select those that still "resonate." Some may not apply to your new space, but may be a vacation or a job or a new love. You can save those for another collage if you want.

- Actually cut out or trim the portion of the picture that you want to keep and set it aside. You may have a great stack of pictures, or just a few, it doesn't matter.

Phase Three: Arrange the pictures on the poster board and glue them down. How they are arranged is a personal choice. Your own ideas will come forward to create just the right constellation.

- Spend some time really looking at what you're creating, and fantasize over the new place: the look and feel of it, the sounds, fragrances and activities you'll enjoy once you're there.

Not only does this activity help create *moving toward* excitement, the process actually works on the basis of the Law of Attraction: the more excitement and joy we experience and can generate about an intention, the more likely it is to become reality. My friend, client and talented creativity coach who introduced me to this process, Shiila Safer and her husband, Dan, have manifested two stunningly different homes using this technique. In each case, the places they were able to find matched their vision to an uncanny degree. I personally did a vision board right after my divorce with only a vague idea of what I wanted my post-divorce life to look like. What grabbed me as I looked through magazines were several pictures:

- A line drawing of a couple having cocktails (I wanted a social life);

- The phrase "change everything;"

- A picture of earth taken from space showing the continent of Asia in the center;

- The words "9.2 million people;"

- A crayon sketch of me standing in front of a crowd with energy moving between us.

Here's what came about within the next three weeks:

- I received an invitation to be the guest speaker on the topic of Feng Shui as the guest of Princess Cruise lines on the Asia portion of an around the world cruise;

- The city of departure for my portion of the cruise was Hong Kong, which at that time boasted a population of 9.2 million people, a fact unknown to me when I made the collage;

- I remembered that the line drawing of the couple I had cut out had been cut away from the larger picture of them on a cruise ship;

- Within that time, I had made an offer on the West Virginia house by selling my Texas home, thereby "changing everything."

The collage process effectively de-emphasizes the logic function of the left-brain and engages the right hemisphere, which allows us to dream without the critic and create like a child at play. We can access joy without our adult voice coming in to spoil the fun! Every client who has used this process has seen or felt the difference this type of creative process allows. Even if all that comes through is choice of colors and style, that one thing can be the spark that builds hope.

Summary and Major Points

1. While a move is rife with reasons to induce stress, it also represents opportunities to:

- Be helpful;

- Be supportive;

- Act with compassion;

- Share memories;

- Re-frame our history; and

- Handcraft the future.

2. By establishing our intentions about how we want to support our parents before the process starts and reaffirming them before each action, we help create the atmosphere of compassion and love.

3. The difference between moving "away from" or "toward" something influences not only day-to-day decisions, but also how quickly the house sells.

4. Working with our families brings up unresolved childhood issues and presents us with an opportunity to resolve or re-script some of them.

5. Thoughts and emotions influence events and relationships.

6. "Every thought has a receiver."

7. Thought re-framing is a process that changes:

- Brain chemistry;

- How we feel; and

- How we relate to others.

8. The must helpful emotions to counteract frustrations are:

- Love;

- Joy;

- Gratitude; and

- Compassion.

9. Discovering and respecting boundaries builds trust and supports the process.

10. Making a collage with your parent is a way you can use creative visualization to move toward excitement.

Suggested Activities

These activities are primarily intended for the children, or others who are managing or assisting with the move. After doing them in that capacity, you might offer the same questions rephrased as appropriate to your parents. This can open dialogue about significant issues and help redirect old patterns and assumptions, making it possible to redirect everyone's energy.

1. Arrange for a few minutes of uninterrupted time and think about how you would like the process of moving your parents to look and feel. Write down your intentions. Be sure to include your husband, wife or children in this process.

2. Identify what you think might be the "landmines" you have to watch out for. Even though others might arise, you can plan alternatives for those emotional obstacles you can identify. Examples might be old childhood patterns, work and time issues, your parent's hearing problem, etc.

3. What negative assumptions are you bringing to the process? List them along with their reframed versions.

4. What are your hopes for the way life will improve for your parents as the result of this move?

7

Selling the House

If you are helping your parents to move, chances are you're also thinking about selling their house. The good news is that many of the things needed for the move are the very things that need to be done to properly present the property to sell quickly and for the highest price. For either process, clearing the clutter, packing up personal items, getting rid of things you are not using, and emotionally releasing the house are essential. But there's more...that's if you want to minimize time on the market AND get the highest price. What follows is a pretty exhaustive inventory of details that can and should be attended to if you want to maximize profit and avoid doing unnecessary repairs. Some of this you may want to hire out or do yourself, but there may be things your parent(s) can do and will want to do to feel more a part of the process.

During my mother's move, my sister and I did the heavy work, helped her make decisions about divesting, met with the realtor, and did a million other smaller tasks. But between visits, Mom had her own list of things she wanted to do and was able to attend to personally and without the time constraints of our visits. She made arrangements for plants she cared about, went through the jewelry she had collected over years of traveling, began sorting through hobby materials and deciding what she was most likely to be able to do at the other end. Yard work was out, quilting was in... So if your folks are able to help, embrace what they can bring to the process, whatever that may be.

Choices

Some families have been faced with the need to get out as quickly as possible. They have chosen to leave all but the most cherished belongings in the house and sell the whole kit and caboodle for auction prices. Others have had more time and accomplished the move and sale more gradually.

Either choice is OK, if it really works for you. The usual scenario is somewhere in the middle, involving adult offspring busy with their own lives and having little time to deal with yet another property, especially in the face of grief.

There are several possible options if indeed you are left with a house filled with decades of belongings, far from your own home. This book focuses primarily on moves where at least one parent is able to participate in some decisions about their belongings, and in most cases is moving to alternative space where a modicum of their treasures can accompany them. Situations involving death, sudden changes in health or lucidity are understandably different. In such cases, there may be neither time nor emotional strength to do all that is necessary to bring a property to its optimum condition.

"Jane" and her siblings, faced with the necessity of moving Dad into a nursing home, met for one long weekend and all six of them and their children blitzed through the house, cleaning, organizing, sorting, putting dibs on things they each wanted and carting off the rest for trash, resale or charity. Before the process started, Dad was urged to make choices about what he wanted to take with him or give to specific family members. After that, he left it up to the kids to make the decisions. They all got along, worked late into the night, went out to eat and got the house emptied, cleaned and listed in the course of four days. I would only recommend this if your folks feel comfortable with being off-site and trusting everyone else with these decisions. To have six people asking them questions, making decisions and carting things off would overwhelm most people, much less an elderly parent. In working with many such clients, I've found that five hours of focus is about maximum, and that only with frequents breaks and shifting of focus.

In my Mom's case, we had a longer lead-time and my sister and I took turns traveling from D.C. and Texas to spend a few days to a week going through things, with Mom having an active voice in every decision. If your parents are able, do everything you can to include them in the process to ensure ownership and reduce the possibility of misunderstandings later. This is more critical than it seems, as there are relationships at stake.

Auctions and Estate Sales

If left with mountains of belongings after family members have made their choices, and quick disposal of the remainder is necessary, one possibility to consider is an estate sale or auction. In either case, there are services that will take care of everything from pricing to transport and storage. I recommend that clients preside over an estate sale only if they really like the process and can emotionally handle their folks' things being sold for bargain basement prices. People expect deals at an estate sale, so this may cover some expenses but I wouldn't expect it to be a moneymaker. Do a mental cost/benefit analysis before making a decision. Consider how much help will be available for setting up, keeping track of money, prices and buyers in addition to the emotional issues.

The option of holding an auction works not only for the contents of the house, but for the house itself. Contrary to popular belief, auctions are not only for distress situations. In some countries they are THE way properties are sold, and even in the U.S., written bid auctions can result in a higher selling price than might come as the result of a traditional sale. You and your parents or family may choose to auction some or all of the belongings as well as the house and land. These should be valued separately, inasmuch as the sale price of the property determines the property taxes to be paid and bundling the two will result in an unrealistically high property value, and therefore a higher tax valuation. This is true whether you choose a traditional sale or an auction, and an experienced buyer or investor will insist on this.

If you're an auction lover, you may already know some of what follows, so feel free to skip ahead. Auctioneers are licensed professionals who hold specialty certifications and can be located by contacting either your state agency or the national associations: National Auctioneers Association (NAA) and National Auctioneers Licensed Law Officials Association (NALLOA). At print time, there were 27 specialties to choose from, ranging from Numismatist and antiques to computer equipment, intellectual property and carnivals. The websites for each of these entities also offer extensive education regarding the auction process.

In addition to being licensed as an Auctioneer, there are individuals licensed to value the personal property you may be offering. Getting the property valued may help you to make the decision to go with an auction or an estate sale. If you decide to take the auction route, the next decision will be whether to have the auction on site, or have the contents moved immediately, stored, and combined with a larger property for auction at a later date. This decision depends on the condition of the physical space where the property is held, time constraints, and the amount of property suitable for auction, all of which the auctioneer can help you determine. In the case of an historical home filled with antiques, having an on site auction can be an advantage.

All of this brings us to the matter of fees. In the traditional real estate sale, the standard commission is 6%, but many realtors are now negotiating commissions and some agencies and independents will offer a fee as low as 1%. It pays to shop, but more important than the commission is whether the realtor knows the area, the level of marketing that will be provided, the number of open houses that will be held, and the reputation of the agent. Selling your own property is advisable only if you are extremely familiar with the process. It helps if you have professional backup for contracts, inspections, etc., feel comfortable with your ability to value the property realistically and not emotionally, and can be "on call" to show the property at a moment's notice. Even if you decide to represent yourself, your willingness to work with a Buyer's Agent will expand your market considerably.

Auction fees and commissions have a wider range of variability, depending on what specific services are being provided. If the auctioneer is valuing, transporting or storing personal property for an offsite auction (SOLE Auction) there may be a separate fee negotiated up front for these services, in addition to a percentage of the sale price. One option for pricing contents is called a Buyer's Premium, where an agreed upon and publicized percentage of the sales price is added to the bid. For example, a Buyer's Premium of 20% on an item sold for a bid of $100 would result in a carryout price of $120.00. Buyer's Premiums can range from 25% to 50%.

You have other options if you can devote a little time to preparing the house. Perhaps your parents are continuing to live in the house while making the necessary preparations for the transition. If you have this opportunity, I recommend the following approach to optimizing your property. By optimizing, I do not mean perfecting. I'm talking about taking the property you have, fixing the obvious and the inexpensive, and presenting it in its best possible light using essentially what you have on hand.

Instructions to the Cook

A lovely book, *Instructions to the Cook: A Zen Master's Lessons on Living a Life That Matters* (Glassman and Fields, 1997) talks about the honor and the challenge faced by the cook in a Buddhist temple. It is the cook's job to prepare the most nutritious and beautifully presented meal possible, make adjustments that were deemed necessary and to see that the assembly feels "at ease." This is the challenge we face with our homes as well. The temple-cook cannot run to the nearest Whole Foods or Safeway to get a little of this and that. In the case of selling our home, we are generally loath to spend a lot of money to make adjustments for others when we wouldn't do it for ourselves. So we optimize, inasmuch as possible by using our creativity and what we have on hand to see that people feel "at ease" and welcome when coming to our home.

In the real estate industry, there is a well-known relationship between days on the market and selling price. Unless your aim is to get out fast and let the house go for whatever you can get for it, the goal is *always* to prepare the property so that it shows at its best before it ever goes on the market and before it is seen by other agents.

Many sellers, anxious to get the process started, will insist that the property be listed and shown as quickly as possible and "see how it goes." After the house fails to sell, only then do they consider getting it in shape: making a few repairs, sprucing it up and having it staged. Such an approach is a mistake because it's very difficult to get prospective buyers or agents back in to see the property once it's been re-done. Worse is the fact that the clock has been ticking and the days-on-the-market have been adding up, all the while knocking the price down. The first question an experienced buyer asks is, "How long has the property been on the market?" Whether it's an investor or first time buyer, everyone knows they can negotiate a better deal (translate "lower price") when the house has been on the market for longer than average.

Roll Up Your Sleeves

So, roll up your sleeves, rev-up the weed eater, drag the cleaning supplies out and get ready to Arrange Your Listing for Success! The tips I'm about to give you have been tried and proven by realtors and sellers alike and come from the above-titled course I've been teaching realtors for many years. This is a compressed version of that eight-hour for-credit course. We'll start with some general guidelines first, followed by specific recommendation for each room.

It's crucial to understand that a prospective buyer makes an emotional decision about the property within about 30 seconds of walking through the front door. Lighting, smells, cleanliness and clutter hit us at the subconscious level and a buyer may never make the connection that their reaction was due to something that can be corrected. Even investors are not immune to these first gut-level judgments about the space, and little can be done at a later date to change that first gestalt response. I've heard buyers spend the next two hours trying to intellectualize why an otherwise perfect house is not right, because they had a negative response to something like a political cartoon, religious messages or symbols, music or cooking odors, etc. Taking care of these things prior to showing can save the sale.

Lighting

Overhead lighting is functional, but it offers little in terms of ambience and appeal. It's the lamps in corners, on side tables, and tucked into bookcases and nooks-and-crannies that really give a room a sense of warmth and invite us to stay. Lamps should be left ON while the house is being shown. It's not enough to have the realtor rush in and turn the lights on after the client arrives. By that time the viewer has already experienced the lack of light and has made the decision that "this is a dark house." Older sellers are loath to leave the lights on because of the sense of waste, and ordinarily I would agree that conserving electricity is a good idea. In the case of a house for sale, however, the increase in utility bills is nothing compared to the money that will be *left on the table* because the buyer thought the house was too dark. Turning on every light in the house will not correct the first visceral response. As a compromise, leave the lights on in all rooms that can be glimpsed from or near the entry. That gives you time to run upstairs and turn on the other lights. But don't take my word for it; try it in your own space. Several of my clients have written to comment that even their husbands commented on the change by noticing how much cozier the home felt.

Clutter

Get rid of it! Nothing says too small, uncared for, neglected, or leaves a more negative impact on the mood of the prospective buyer. The underlying assumption is: if this much neglect is evident when the house is being shown, imagine what cannot be seen. The truth is, clutter creates allergies, fatigue, bugs, mold, depression, frustration, alienation, and myriad other problems, none of which support a sale. Finally, clearing it will put you well on your way to moving!

In terms of selling a house, clutter is a little different from the normal day-to-day evidence of living in a house. When a property is on the market, it is competing with model homes where no expense has been spared to furnish, stage and landscape. The purpose is to create the fantasy of living a beautiful-people, carefree lifestyle, "if I lived here." Clutter immediately takes the bloom off an otherwise beautifully put-together home. For a house on the market, clutter can take the form of:

- Personal belongings left on the counter;

- Medications and medical paraphernalia left in full view;

- Evidence of pet hair, odors, unkempt food trays;

- Clothing left around;

- Disorganized garage, closets, and overfull storage;

- An abundance of gadgets, knick-knacks, family pictures, souvenirs.

Getting rid of the clutter has a mobilizing and comforting effect on everyone I've worked with. A letter I received after a de-cluttering session from Sharon in Austin is characteristic of the feelings people experience:

"How exuberant, exciting, and healthy I feel. I have even stopped taking medication I had depended on for so long simply because I don't feel the need for them or at least not as often as before. I feel so much more relaxed and alive and excited to get up and start each day. I just feel like a brand new person."

Odors

Many people are sensitive to tobacco odor, pet hair and dander, sweet perfumes in candles and air-sprays, and certain cleaning substances. In addition to being offensive, there is another aspect of odors that can be subconsciously related to regional or ethnicity prejudices or other associations. Remove the source of the odor if possible and buy or rent a high quality air purifier. If the source of the odor is present throughout the listing time, keep the purifier running. If the odors are intense and do not respond to normal remedies, I recommend you call in a professional service. Having bought and sold many properties for investment and personal residences, as well as having owned and managed multi-family properties, I've personally had to remove carpet fouled by pet urine, chemically sanitize the foundation, and seal it before replacing the carpet. Simply eliminating the odor prior to showing can avoid this thought ever coming to mind for the buyer. When odors are present, there is the assumption (often correct) that the remedy will be extremely expensive. Because the sense of smell is one of the first to be impacted with aging, aging parents my be oblivious or have acclimated to even strong odors in their home. Therefore, they may not be a good judge of whether or not the odor has been eliminated. If in doubt, have a third party do a sniff-test.

Curb Appeal

Home searches have changed over the years as more people are using the Internet to locate and screen properties before anyone ever drives by. Ultimately, however, someone is going to physically look at the property and that first impression will either entice prospective buyers in through the front door or send them running. Here's the short version of sprucing up the curb-appeal.

- Mow, edge, weed and re-sod brown spots in the lawn;

- Replace or remove dead shrubs;

- Have shrubs *properly* trimmed—no flat-topping!

- Repair ragged-looking fences and driveways;

- Prune trees if obscuring the view of the house from the street;
- House numbers should be clearly visible and attractive;
- Replace or paint sad-looking mailboxes;
- Clean exterior lighting fixtures and make sure they work;
- Remove clutter, toys, and trashcans from the front yard;
- Remove old cars, trailers, and debris;
- Repair or replace screens and clean windows visible from the street.

Politics, Religion, and Other Touchy Subjects

Everyone knows deep inside that these things shouldn't make a difference when buying a property; they belong to the seller and are not a part of the structure or suitability of the property. Right? Technically, yes; emotionally, NO! Even the most broad-minded, egalitarian individual has SOME little piece of viscera that responds to these emotionally loaded topics and it may be so submerged that it would never rationally be a part of any deal.

Carefully, with your parent, edit the home for books, artwork, refrigerator comics, magazines and anything left out for public consumption. It doesn't mean you have to hide ethnicity, but it does mean that it shouldn't be the first thing someone notices about the property. Your parent, the seller, has no way of knowing the history, emotional baggage, preferences, prejudices or predispositions of those wandering through their home. If things are left in view, ask, "Is this worth losing a sale over?"

In some parts of the country, hunting is considered a divine right. Trophies are displayed with pride and animal skins adorn the floors and walls. On quite a few occasions I've been called in to consult with clients who have felt it's important to show the property as a "hunter's paradise," and have steadfastly refused to pack away their trophies. In one city home I stepped into the family room boasting a cowhide on the floor, the full horsehide from a pet named Honey on the love seat, and a cowhide drink coaster next to each seat. I'm not talking about standard leather furniture; that doesn't seem to trigger the same reactions. It was the full bearskin rug with the open mouthed black bear in the guest room door that really pushed people over the edge. The sellers didn't remove the skins, and the house has not sold as of this printing. Another open gallery type home boasted twenty trophy heads—all of them staring at guests as they stepped across the threshold. Reluctant at first, the owner took them down when he realized he was cutting out the majority of his market. The house sold for the asking price shortly thereafter.

Consider that one man's paradise is another's prison. Every political statement, animal head, religious affiliation you display can dramatically reduces the size of your buyer pool.

The rule-of-thumb for cabinets, closets and pantries is to have them no more than two-thirds full, to give the impression that there is room to grow. Your folks will be getting rid of clothing they no longer wear anyway, and this is an excellent opportunity. If some closets are packed and others empty, put off-season clothing in an empty closet. Since some parents will be moving to an altogether different climate to be nearer family, thinning out for geographical reasons might make the process easier. If this is the case, we can reduce the fear of never returning by keeping a few pieces for anticipated trips back to see friends (even if *we* believe that will never happen). Simply getting rid of out-of-date mixes, spices and canned goods can clear significant space in pantries. Organizing foods by group and using turntables give an impression of order and actually make life easier while continuing to use the kitchen. Here are a few additional tips for creating space in closets and cabinets:

- Keep floors clear except for neatly organized shoes, etc.;

- Vertical shoe storage can be inexpensive and creates order;

- Minimize the size and number of items stored on shelves over the hanging racks;

- Look at storage ideas in Chapter 10 (Unpacking and Settling In) for more ideas on maximizing storage. Some expenses are worth the effort when selling a home, even if you can't take the items with you.

Specific Room and Area Recommendations for Your Parents

Front door entry

- Remove clutter from front door area;
- Clean and repaint front door if necessary;
- Clean brass-work and door hardware;
- Repair or oil locks so they work easily;
- If seasonal, add flowers or live plants in entry;
- Trim overgrown vines;
- Sweep away spider webs often;
- Weed and/or mulch flowerbeds near front door;
- Keep area swept.

Foyer

- Should feel open and be well lighted;
- All rooms seen from entry should be well arranged and have lights on;
- Area rug adds warmth;
- Eliminate odors (pet, tobacco, mold, cooking) with an air purifier. Rent one if necessary;
- DO NOT USE SWEET CANDLES or POPOURRI!

Bathrooms

- Keep toilet lids down and toilets immaculately clean;
- Repair, clean or replace faucets if necessary. The decorative inserts can be replaced inexpensively to make faucets look new;
- Use lime away or vinegar (as appropriate) to remove hard water deposits and scale;
- Clean tubs and showers and glass doors with soap-scum remover and polish tiles with a towel;

- Remove mold in tub and showers, re-caulk if necessary;

- Replace old shower curtains with one that has a neutral pattern, and leave half open or fully drawn for softness;

- Use fluffy new towels (you can take them with you) for updating;

- If you have a garden tub, stage it with a basket of luxury bath products and candles to create a spa fantasy;

- Leave a nightlight on in interior bathrooms;

- A small lamp with low-wattage bulb left on instead of harsh overhead lighting creates ambiance;

- Large bathrooms can use an area rug for elegance (as opposed to standard bath mats);

- Clear personal products and daily use items from counters (or put in baskets to hide);

- Clear all cabinets to 2/3 full;

- Fold linens and stack neatly to impart sense of space and extra storage;

- REMOVE toilet plungers and cleaning wands (no need to suggest problems);

- Replace valves if toilet "runs" after flushing.

Kitchen

- Pantry should be no more than 2/3 full. Pack items away if necessary;

- Reduce under-sink items to essentials;

- Bleach sinks if stained;

- Clean and polish faucets, replace washers if leaky;

- Clean oven and replace burner pans if stained or crusted;

- Clear counter tops of all but essentials. Put toaster ovens, broilers and the like under counter for showing;

- Use a bowl of fresh lemons to freshen the air naturally and create an image of health and well-being;

- Clean oven hood and any appliances of oily buildup;

- Replace low-wattage fixtures with highest wattage bulbs possible to optimize lighting. Replace yellowed light covers;

- Pack away recipe books and knick-knacks, remove notes and magnets from refrigerator door;

- Remove or replace soiled kitchen rugs;

- Freshen paint if necessary and wipe down or oil cabinets;

- Keep only needed cooking utensils, dinnerware, etc.;

- Remember the 2/3 full rule and pack everything else away;

- If you're going to do the fresh-baked-cookies thing, BAKE them! Cookie fragranced spray smells are detected as fake and are a turn-off.

Bedrooms

- Remove desks, computers, and workout equipment: they imply there's not enough room in the house (can also interfere with sleep);

- Each side of the bed should have a bedside table and lamp (suggests this is a home for couples and relationships);

- Clear tops of dressers, chests of drawers of personal items and clutter;

- Remove family pictures;

- Remove items from under the bed (suggests insufficient storage);

- The Master Bedroom is the most important. Stage it by turning down the covers, standing the pillows against the headboard, use your best linens to make it feel like the best bed-and-breakfast, which suggests comfort, intimacy and pampering.

Family Room

- Arrange according to the suggestions in Chapter 9. When possible, position a group that feels like open-arms when you walk into the room. Avoid having the couch with its back facing to you when you walk into the room. It says "Private. Keep Out," the antithesis of the feeling you want to engender when you're selling the house;

- Casually scatter a few pillows and/or an afghan in complimentary colors to suggest time to curl up and read or watch movies;

- Establish a reading corner, if there's room. Place a comfy chair with a side table, lamp, throw and an open book for the idea that there will be TIME to read and reflect;

- A game left open and set up on the coffee table suggests family time, something most families have difficulty creating.

Rooms set up in this way beckon us to stay a while and entertain the kids who come to look at the house with their parents. The longer you can engage a prospective buyer, the more likely it is they'll make an offer. A home on the market MUST engage the buyer emotionally. Realtors will confirm that many a contract has been written on houses that didn't meet the logical criteria because the buyer identified with the emotions elicited by the property. My first experience with this was on the occasion that I made a slight adjustment in my own living room when my oldest son was about sixteen and, by his own admission, couldn't care less about anything beyond the location of the couch, TV and the refrigerator. He considered himself pretty macho, and was already doing volunteer firefighter duty at a local fire department. I kept all of the pieces in their same location relative to each other and had only changed the angle of the whole constellation about 15 degrees, so it wasn't at all obvious that anything had been moved. When he came home that day he literally dropped his book bag, sucked in a deep breath and said "Wow, it feels so good in here!" Anyone out there who has parented teenage sons will appreciate how stunning such an unsolicited statement is! He didn't say "Oh, you moved the furniture," or "Oh, it looks different, what'd you do?" It's the *feeling and sense of comfort* we're going after.

Office

Arrange desks according to the guidelines in Chapter 9, with the desk in the Power Position whenever possible. If that's not practical, position it to face out into the room with a wall behind the desk chair.

- Clear the surface of the desk of all but essentials;
- Mail can be put in a basket or in/out box;
- Pack enough books to leave some open space in bookcases and alternate with a few plants or art pieces for an updated look;
- Remove EVERYTHING from the knee space under the desk;
- If there's room, create a reading nook with a lamp;
- If you have an extra, place a lamp on the corner of the desk and leave it on for showing;
- Pack up office supplies that are not in use to create room in closets;
- Bundle and hide electronics cords. If you have cords hanging behind the exposed front of a desk, bundle them and use a floor plant to hide. In addition to camouflaging the cords, a plant brings life, energy and class. Silk plants are fine, but keep them dusted.

Laundry Room

This is a frequently neglected room, but because we spend so much time there and it's such a luxury to have one, doll it up a little. Don't be afraid to hang artwork, use a wonderful color and otherwise treat it like a respected part of the house.

- Put cleaning supplies and detergents behind doors;
- If there are open cabinets, consider placing smaller containers in baskets so they don't look cluttered;
- Remove empty hangers, piles of clothing, etc.;
- Use attractive hampers (wicker, straw, etc.), which can sit on top of the washer and dryer.

Garage

I'm always surprised when clients ask me, "Does the garage count?" In a word, YES! The garage tends to be used as the family landfill and it has just about the same appeal when it's neglected and cluttered. It's imperative that you be able to park a car INSIDE the garage—what a concept!

- Painting the garage adds perceived value;

- Increase vertical storage. Tube-construction, vinyl shelves are inexpensive, easily moved with you and can be configured to match the space and the items to be stored;

- Items to be kept can be grouped and stored in large plastic bins, which can be easily moved when the time comes;

- Pegboard can add value because rakes, hoses, sports gears etc. can be hung neatly and made more accessible;

- Clean floor of oil spills and stains. Epoxy paint adds value;

- Lawn gear that will not accompany you on the move can be given to places like Habitat for Humanity, sold cheaply or included with the house;

- Since chemicals cannot be moved in the moving van, consider offering them to neighbors or storing them neatly in boxes or on shelves for the new owners;

- Old paint cans with current house paint colors can be disposed of after noting the paint color, brand and formula in a notebook as a courtesy for the new owners;

- Remove items that emit strong chemical or insecticide odors.

Summary and Major Points

1. Many of the things we do to get ready for a down-sizing move are the same things that need to be done to properly present the house to sell quickly and for the highest price:

- De-clutter;

- Pack up personal items;

- Get rid of things you're no longer using;

- Emotionally release the property.

2. Give the process as much lead time as possible.

3. If left with many belongings after everyone has had their say, consider an estate sale or auction.

4. Auction or sale prices should separate the value of the property from the value of the contents.

5. The selling price of the house, land and other buildings on the land determine the property taxes.

6. Auctioneers are licensed professionals and have specialty certifications.

7. The value of the belongings can be determined by individuals who specialize in that area.

8. Staging the house, making strategic decisions about presentation and repairs will help reduce time on the market and maximize selling price.

9. Attend to room-by-room details to trigger the potential buyer's emotional connection to the property:

- Lighting;

- Clutter;

- Odor;

- Curb appeal;

- Removal of political or religious items;

- Storage;

- Room arrangement.

Suggested Activities

These activities are useful even if you, the helper, are the only one who participates. It's certainly desirable to have your parent engaged in the process, but if they are resistant, these ideas can serve as a guide for productive conversations.

1. Talk with your parent(s) about their desires for divesting of belongings they no longer need. Determine in general terms what their desires are regarding giving belongings to other family members or charities, having an estate sale, or selling certain items via an auction. Make a note of their feelings and any specific items that hold special importance.

2. Offer your parents the opportunity to read this chapter, or discuss it with them to determine what items they feel they can or would like to handle. Even minor participation can create ownership and a sense of purpose. It can also reduce the list of details for which you and other helpers are responsible.

3. List the items you can take care of when readying the house for sale.

4. List activities you will require help with.

5. List the names of friends, relatives or professionals you might call upon to help with tasks you will not be handling.

8

Streamlining and Packing

Many of us at this stage of life are moving into smaller, more efficient or manageable homes, but even if that's not the case, no one wants to pack and pay to move things that no longer serve them. The same process that guides our parents' paring-down process prepares them for a much smoother and less costly move. If there is enough lead-time before the move, my approach is to start the streamlining process as soon as you both begin thinking about their move. The more lead-time you have, the more thorough, relaxed and creative the process can be.

- Every moment you and your parent spend de-cluttering and making conscious decisions about what they take will save you time, money and frustration at both ends of the move;

- Decisions about what to take are predicated on the intentions you set for the Nine Life Domains: *Health, Activities, Spirituality, Family, Finance, Extensions, Relationship, Creativity, Travel/Help*;

- With each item, the question for your parent(s) to consider is: "Does this support my life goals for the next stage?" If the answer is NO, perhaps you can help them make the decision to let it go. But, in the end, it's their decision.

Streamlining might start with things that are not actively used on a daily basis: books, tools, clothing, and the contents of bathroom cabinets. When you've picked a starting point, group *like with like*. When you can see how much or how many of a specific category you have, it's easier to see what can go. Once they discover they have eight pairs of black slacks, knowing which ones can go is faster and easier. Consolidating cosmetics, cleaning supplies, shoes, tools, toys, books, etc. also allows them to determine if the new space will accommodate their current inventory, giving them a better idea of just how much they need to let go. Once it's been determined what stays, some thought can be given to the type of storage they will need, plan for, or create.

Now What?

Every organizing project, whether you've seen it on TV, in a book, a class or a neighbor's house uses three basic categories: YES, NO, and I DON'T KNOW.

Question	YES!	NO!
Do I LOVE it?	Organize	Recycle
Does it FIT?	Store it	Charity
Does it WORK??	Keep or recycle	Resale or repair
DO I use it?	Keep it	Throw away Garage sale

Making the Decision

Keeping in mind your intentions in the Nine Life Domains, consider whether there is still a match between each item how it continues to fit in your life.

- **With each item,** the person moving must ask the question:
  - "Does this support my life goals for the **current stage**?" If yes, ask the next set of questions. If no, let it go. If the move is not immediate, keep these items active until closer to the time.
  - Does it support my life goals for the **next** stage? If yes, go to the next level. If no, let it go.

- **Separate the decision** of whether the item will be discarded from the question of where it will find a new home. Too often, a decision is made to keep something that has no further use, simply because we can't decide where it will go. Once the decision to let something go is made, put it with other discards until a final destination is found. Putting a little distance between these decisions is more productive, faster and less stressful.

- **More Useful Questions to Ask Your Parent(s):**
  - **Do you LOVE IT?** Things we truly love support us emotionally and spiritually. Keep it even if it's just to look at.

o **What's important to you about this?** This question unearths the real meaning of the item and calls for a conscious decision. It protects us from keeping things through default.

o **How will it be used at the new place?** If you find them trying to figure out a use for it and they don't love it, I encourage leaving it behind.

o **Does it fit NOW?** As we mature, bodies change and styles we wore two or three sizes ago may not fit our new body. It's a good way to justify letting go of clothing — and it has the advantage of being true!

o **How many of these (items) do** you **realistically need?** If there are duplicates, is there a reason to keep extras?

Strategies

- **By categories:** do major categories throughout the house. For example, if you're doing clothing, go to every closet and dresser, group items by type (pants, shirts, blouses) and determine how many there are in each category. Do they fit, do they have matching pieces, how many do you need, etc. Pack those you will not need until after the move. Do the same with other categories like medications, etc.

- **By room:** go through each room systematically, starting with the rooms least used, sort by category and ask the above questions. If you know there are other items in like categories, box them to put with other like items before you pack, unless you know they will go into a specific room with other items in a group. Pack as you go when possible. Label according to the guidelines listed later in this chapter.

Boxes of Inherited Items or Memorabilia

Going through one box at a time, separate out items that represent the **most** salient **positive** memories of the events "housed" in the box. Options for managing items that are truly important range from keeping the most important ones in an artistic shadow-box frame or keepsake box, to sharing them with others in a scrapbook, or having a family gathering to remember and divide the items. During this process, if you're doing it with parents, take advantage of the opportunity to let them talk about people and events. I learned so much about my mother's life while going through old documents. My father, long deceased, became part of that process while we revisited papers going back to the end of WWII, and we were able to re-experience his sense of humor and mischievousness. This time can be a true gift and can build bridges to improve relationships.

Discarded Items have many possible destinations:

- Family or friends;
- Schools, museums, libraries;
- Charity;
- Consignment centers;
- Auction;
- Personal Garage sale;
- Churches' tag sales;
- Internet sales: e-Bay, Craig's List.

If you get stuck and don't know where to turn next, you can always use the Quick-Throw cheat sheets. The Quick-Throw lists that follow are guilt-free. Most of the things can be thrown away, but some things like craft items and games can be given to charities.

Use Your Intuition!

This little technique is a great shortcut to the kind of mental gymnastics we find ourselves in when trying to decide what to keep or pass on. Believe it or not, we have some emotional relationship or energetic response to everything that has made its way into our homes. Everyone I know has had the experience of walking into a house or business and immediately sensing something either "spooky" or wonderful about the place. We feel that about people too, and it's often that inner compass that steers us away from danger.

The good news is that we can feel it about things as well. When I met a new neighbor for the first time, she invited me into her home and was showing me around. As we went into the study my eyes feel on an old book and I picked it up. The moment I touched it I was embraced by an irrepressible sense of joy and a huge grin spread across my face. My new friend asked what I was smiling about and I responded with "This book feels so good—it makes me happy to touch it!" She was a little shocked by the answer and asked me to tell her more. She then explained that as a little boy, her husband had received the book from his father who was known as a wonderful, kind man. Her husband had spent many summer hours of his childhood propped up in a tree, reading this book and I'd felt those feelings when I handled it.

It's easiest to identify those feelings with people we've met, so try this out by standing in front of pieces of inherited furniture or a few belongings received from friends or family. If this is a totally alien concept for you, skip ahead and try the exercise at the end of this chapter.

The feeling you get when walking into a house or picking up an object is your intuition and it bypasses the logical mind, going straight to the heart of the matter—how things and people make you feel. Most students are surprised to find that at least a few people, about whom they thought they would have good feelings, triggered a negative response.

The goal is to surround yourself with only those things that you really love, or at least those that are really useful. Obviously, you can't throw out the tax return just because it makes you feel bad, but with the exception of legal and financial documents, you have a choice. Clients tell me this has saved them hours of time and frustration and helped them feel really good about the choices they made. It works better for some things than for others. We can usually sense how we felt wearing certain clothes and what memorabilia evokes. If you're really neutral about something, consider letting it go unless there are other compelling reason to keep it. One way to get in tune with intuition is to toss a coin. "Heads I keep it, tails I toss it." Say it comes up tails, and the emotional response is disappointment. Then you go with the feeling and keep it. If the feeling is more like relief, then you go with the coin and toss it.

Quick-Throw Reference

Home Office

- Information you already know;
- Outdated catalogs ("Keep the source/purge the paper");

- Stationary you no longer use: keep a copy for your history file;
- Old financials (beyond retention date);
- Early drafts of creative writing;
- Magazines past one year unless special (can cut and file article).

Traditional Office

- Old magazines/articles/books;
- Old research material (keep the source/toss the paper);
- Duplicates of documents;
- Early drafts;
- Product solicitations;
- Supplies that are bulky and that you don't use.

Household Files

- Junk mail;
- Old grocery receipts and other non-useful receipts;
- Expired coupons and invitations;
- Old greeting cards unless they're REALLY special;
- Out of date schedules;
- Check books over six years old;
- Old maps;
- Expired warranties and policies;
- Canceled checks—except those needed for tax purposes;
- Old catalogs;
- Poor quality pictures;
- Business cards from people you don't remember;
- Unread magazines past three months old;
- Articles/clippings you haven't read in five years;

- Instructions on items you no longer use;
- Old pet tags.

Garages and Attics

- Mildewed bedding, clothing, furniture, rugs, etc.;
- Dried out paint and old chemicals (the city has a toxic waste drop for these);
- Broken garden equipment and hoses;
- Rusty nails, tools and equipment;
- Broken tools, garden pots;
- Old newspapers, magazines, college notebooks (are you really going to use these?);
- Receipts going back seven years or more (check with accountant);
- Obsolete baby equipment;
- Broken electronics equipment and SMALL appliances;
- Gift boxes, used wrapping paper, old greeting cards;
- Broken furniture (with no antique value).

Bathrooms

- Expired medications (keep list of names/doctors if you must);
- Half used and abandoned bottles of anything (shampoo, conditioner, etc.);
- Twisted, leaking, mangled tubes;
- Teensy-weensy pieces of old soap;
- Old nail polish you no longer like;
- Rusty personal care items (tweezers, nail clippers, scissors);
- Duplicate hair accessories: blow dryer, curlers, curling iron (You might put these in a travel pouch and keep with suitcases);
- Worn out bandages (stretched ace wraps, etc.);

- Out of use or sample size cosmetics, perfumes and such (Women's shelters, the State School love these);

- Frayed and ragged towels (retire to Goodwill or a centralized rag bin);

- **Travel sizes:** save a few for a travel case that you keep ready to go, or put aside a few for a guest bath.

Packing Up

A lot of time can be saved and angst avoided by packing as you go. Once you've decided what you'll keep fore the long haul, decide what you can live without in the short term and start packing. If you start early, you can avoid the costly proposition of having professional packers do it for you. If you are physically able and want to make your unpacking on the other end logical, orderly and more fun, DO YOUR OWN PACKING!

First, you get to pack based on the way you've organized. Packing by category will simplify unpacking and settling in at your destination and save you days of anguish. Second, not only are professional packers expensive, their job is to pack your belongings *safely*, not to *organize* them. As a consequence, the oddest things are packed together, and that can make unpacking sheer chaos.

Recently, I have helped a number of clients move into a very upscale retirement community and many have hired "professional" packers. There are differences among many companies and service personnel, and the relocation industry is no different.

In general, it is NOT the job of the packer to make decisions about what to pack with what, other than common sense would allow. In other words, they generally won't pack a cast iron pot on top of crystal, but most will pack anything they find in a room together with other things found in that room, whether or not they logically go together. For example, I've found desk supplies mixed in with toothpaste and pet supplies. If you were packing, you'd logically pack desk supplies together with any belongings that went with that desk, but you'd pass on packing pet toys and toothpaste with them.

In one instance, I'd been present to help a client with other things on packing day and took off a wrist brace, only to discover it had been packed in one of many boxes with no labels other than "office." I bought a new brace and found the old one a week later.

In the same move, the client had asked that her computer be packed in such a way that she could locate it first, to be able to set up her office upon arrival. Since there were two offices in the home from which they moved, and there were twelve generically labeled "office" boxes, it didn't help that none were specified with COMPUTER. We happened upon the box a week later. These packers charged an inordinate amount of money to pack, and made the move far more of a hassle than it should have been.

I've unpacked for others whose belongings were very well packed and labeled. But in each case, the expense was significantly inflated because of the sheer amount of packing material used to avoid liability. I've un-wrapped a thumb-sized wooden knick-knack rolled into a ball of paper the size of a volleyball. Not much economy in that. It really is a trade off. If you do end up needing the services of packers, get references, and ask questions about language fluency, training and employment history.

If You Are Doing the Packing

- First and foremost, decide ahead of time concerning how devastated you would be if a particular item was lost of destroyed. Make other arrangements for key objects. Add to this items you will want IMMEDIATELY upon arrival: telephone? laptop? active medications? pet box? Take these with you in the car, have a friend help, or make other secure arrangements.

- Economize by finding USED moving boxes and packing materials!. Contact nearby retirement communities, realtors and recycling centers to capture supplies that others are off-loading. If you have to buy boxes, many movers and box companies will sell used ones at a vastly reduced price.

- Separate the things you'll need immediately at your destination so they don't get accidentally packed or lost in the chaos. Get out a suitcase or WELL MARKED boxes and put things in as you think of them to avoid forgetting them when things get really frenzied. Segregate them from the rest of the boxes and let the mover know you'd like them loaded last. *Last loaded* translates to *first off* at destination.

- Computer files should be backed up, especially if the hard drive is going on the van. In the extreme case that it is lost or damaged, you'll still have the data and your peace of mind.

- If you are taking live plants, be sure they are well watered and bagged to avoid their leaking or dumping in transit. They will not be insured in transit, so expect the possibility that they'll suffer from climate changes and lack of sunlight.

- In general, organize for packing with an idea of how you'd want to find things at the other end. Unpacking will be made easier if you pack things in categories: like with like or categories that make sense to YOU.

> The exception to this is the use of towels, pillows, bedding etc. as packing material. It saves space and money spent on packing materials.

- Use Zip-lock bags of various sizes to pack smaller items as a group. I use big zip-locks to keep everything from specific desk drawers together, and label which drawer they came from. It saves me from having to start from scratch at the other end.

- I know this seems obvious, but LABEL EVERY BOX with:

  o Room it GOES to at destination. It saves time if you're paying movers by the hour and keeps you from having to move it again when you get there. One client uses the half-inch stick-on dots used for office files. She uses a different color for every room it will go in, and puts one on each side of the box. On moving day, at the destination, she puts a colored dot on the door to the room to tell movers where the box goes.

  o List major items in the box, i.e., New Mexico pottery packed in green comforter, travel book, files from top left desk drawer. Remember that room designations, storage and locations of items will be different at your new place so be especially conscious of categorizing and labeling based on new designations and not current placement.

- o Set aside chemicals that stay with the house, before items are packed. Insurance carriers prevent movers from transporting toxic or flammable substances.

- Pack seasonal clothes together and label them so you can unpack the ones in current use first.

- Use suitcases, coolers, and other empty bags and containers as moving boxes, remembering to label them.

- If possible, put completed, labeled boxes in one room, keeping space open in the rest of the house for getting around. The more order you can maintain while packing up, the greater your sanity will be.

- Designate an area to place things you're going to give away and label it as such. Remember that you don't have to know where it's going until later. Doing this protects unwanted items from being packed by well-meaning friends.

- If you're making a local move, avoid the assumption that you can take things over piecemeal. It's still easier to pack everything, and have it moved all at once.

- Have everything packed BEFORE your movers come. Have items you're taking with you isolated so they don't get put on the truck.

- Save the vacuum cleaner and a few cleaning supplies till last. While movers are there you can be vacuuming the rooms. When Mom made her last move, I cleaned while movers moved. By the time they closed the doors to the van, we were finished with the house. When things were quiet, I spent the last few minutes saying goodbye to the house while Mom said goodbye to her neighbors. (Chapter 12 offers some ideas on rituals to help with saying farewell and moving forward.)

Attics and Underneath the House

Be aware that moving companies WILL NOT enter these areas to move your belongings. Have them emptied by someone else prior to moving day.

Movers and Fees

There are two basic approaches to moving estimates: hourly and by the pound. Long distance movers bid by the pound and they are typically very good at making their estimates, but you have to know AHEAD of time what you're taking to go this route and get a fixed bid. The fixed bid can be a little higher than the actual weight bid so talk to your mover about these options. Generally, the fixed bid option will guarantee your move not to exceed a certain amount, with a reduction if the weight is less than estimated. Another route is actual weight, but without a firm prior estimate you could be in for a huge surprise if you forget items or add items at the last minute.

Many local moves are hourly and this can be an eye-opener. Because it's hourly, you are at the mercy of the skill and experience level of the movers. Skill and training in moving large items and using ergonomic equipment and carrying techniques make a significant difference in cost. One of my clients received a bid from a well-known local company for a six-hour move requiring one truck. Inefficient loading resulted in an eighteen hour move with two trucks. The movers were cheerful and helpful throughout the move, but the cost was exorbitant. The clients ended up paying for all the waiting time to receive a second truck and needless to say it was an unsatisfactory experience.

The bottom line is to check out your options thoroughly and start scheduling early since some seasons are busier than others. Late spring after school lets out and early fall, just before school starts are the busiest times of the year.

Summary and Major Points

1. Streamlining before packing saves time, money and frustration at the destination.

2. Use the Nine Life Domains to help you determine preferences about what will be useful in your new life.

3. Group like-with-like before discarding, and keep together when packing.

4. Every decision is basically:

- Keep;
- Throw;
- I Don't Know.

5. Isolate the decision to discard an item from where it will go after discarding.

6. Other useful questions to help with a decision to keep or discard:

- Do you LOVE IT?
- What's important to you about this?
- How will you use it in your new place?
- Does it fit NOW?
- How many of these do you realistically need?

7. Work strategies:

- By category;
- By room.

Suggested Activities

1. With a friend or partner, make a list of twenty-five people you've come in contact with over the years. Write down the first names that come to mind—it can be the grocery clerk, boss, family member—even just the word "plumber" if you can't recall the name. Do it fast and without spending a lot of time thinking about whom you'll list. When you're through, trade lists with your partner and have him call out each name (in random order) and allow time to sense the feeling you get in your body when you hear the name. You may feel a lift in your spirits, a knot in your stomach, sadness, a jolt of anger or tenderness. By identifying the way positive or negative emotions feel in your body, you can generalize this information to the sense you get when holding items. This is a shortcut to help you decide what no longer supports you.

2. Make a list of the things you want immediately when you arrive

- Clothing;

- Computer;

- Medications;

- Hobby supplies;

- Bedding;

- Art work;

- School supplies;

- Tools;

- Address file.

3. What things do you want to take in the car with you?

- Phone;

- Hard drive;

- Laptop;

- Medications;

- Pet bed;

- Overnight bag.

9

Seeing the Big Picture

When I was a new mother in the hospital after giving birth to my firstborn, I was awakened from a sound sleep one morning by a nurse's announcement over the public address system: "THEY'RE COMING—READY OR NOT!" The next sounds were those of the nursery doors clanging open and the cacophony of screaming babies interspersed with the rattle of bassinette wheels racing down the halls delivering hungry babies to nursing mothers. Anyone who has nursed their baby knows the mixed joy and fear for those first few days. Panic and excitement balanced by pain and pleasure!

Panic might well be what you are feeling at the prospect of being the midwife for the birthing of this next stage of life for your parents. And THEY will come, READY or not, but fortunately, it's just the movers. Will you be ready? I mentioned the idea of sketching a floor plan with the approximate locations of beds, couches and desks, but where should they go to create the most comfortable, welcoming and functional placement? (Read on...)

The way we arrange a room can make the difference between recuperative rest and fitful sleep, creativity or inability to focus, congenial conversation or argument. So it behooves us to plan ahead and pay attention to where we put the bed, the couch or the desk. It's not just about where it fits! It's about how it feels and how *we* feel when we're using those things.

The colors we use can cause us to feel happy or sad, energized or sleepy, calm or anxious. Lighting can do the same, as can sound. Every element of the space contributes to our overall sense of safety, well-being, productivity, creativity, and sense of home.

Some of the information we have about what feels comfortable comes from the ancient practice of Feng Shui mentioned in Chapter Three's discussion of Life Domains and balance. Some of the recommendations for placement come from anecdotal evidence gathered from experiences spanning thousands of years and numerous continents and cultures. Others come from the world of ergonomics, psychology and just plain common sense. Having applied the principles discussed and diagramed in this chapter hundreds of times, and having both witnessed and heard about the results, I can attest to improved sleep patterns, mood changes, enhanced communication, and soaring productivity and creativity. Add to this what we know about the physiological effects and emotional impact of color, light and sound, and we have valuable tools for creating a space that embraces you with comfort, productivity and psychological fit.

Let's start with some basic arrangement guidelines. If special needs are present, as with the use of walkers or wheelchairs, diminished vision or hearing, Parkinson's Disease or Alzheimer's, there is additional information to be found about specific challenges in Chapter 13. The diagrams in this chapter will help you develop a template for the larger design. This process will help you decide not only where things will fit, but assist with making decisions about what pieces of furniture should go or stay. Additionally, this template will guide the movers in placing the large pieces at the moment of moving in.

Chapter 10 includes these guidelines, but with an eye toward filling in the details, adding storage, hanging pictures, etc. Think of this chapter as providing the framework, with the embellishments and practical details following in Chapter 10.

Bedrooms

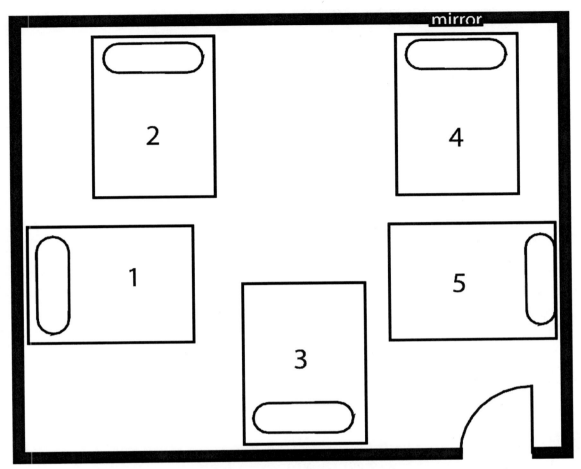

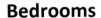

Diagram 1: Bed Placement

Since the primary focus for the bedroom is privacy, the ideal placement for a bed is one that affords the largest view of the room AND a view of the door. Seeing the door does not mean being in LINE with the door, which results in a sense of vulnerability. We are at our most vulnerable state while sleeping, and we depend on feeling safe to be able to fully rest. Part of the psyche is always on guard if we feel ill-at-ease (even at a subconscious level) and we may wake frequently during the night or face the morning feeling exhausted, even after a full night of sleep.

- Diagram 1 shows preferred bed placements, with Position 1 being *best* and Position 5 being worst. One and two are about the same and the choice can be made depending on other pieces of furniture (bedside tables, dressers, chest-of-drawers) and windows.

- Position 3 doesn't afford a view of the door and can result in our feeling subconsciously "at risk" even if at a conscious level we feel safe. I've seen this placement cause a feeling of dis-ease in the room, as well as interfering with sleep and intimacy. If you MUST put the bed in this position, consider a mirror positioned where you can see the door when looking at the mirror while reclining in the bed. (See diagram).

- Positions 4 and 5 can seriously interfere with sleep or rest, leaving the occupant feeling exposed.

Bedside tables

Each person should have a bedside table for both the obvious functional reasons (lighting, reading material, medications, tissue, etc.) and for symbolic reasons, to support the idea of equality in the relationship. They don't have to match, but it's important that they feel roughly equal in relative weight, size, and importance. A significant imbalance not only affects our sense of aesthetics, but can also suggest unequal importance or value in the relationship. Height differences can be counter-balanced by the effective use of artwork, lamps and accessories.

Mirrors

These can play havoc with restful sleep for any number of reasons. First, mirrors can reflect light coming in from the outside, or frighten us when we get up in the middle of the night and see our image. Before we're fully awake and realize the image is ours and not that of an intruder, our adrenalin has shot through the roof and it's hard to get back to sleep. A room full of mirrors or lined with mirrored doors feels like we're on exhibition on in the House of Mirrors! (I don't know about you, but the idea of seeing myself in triplicate dragging out of bed with messed hair, smeared mascara and looking my age doesn't inspire "Good Morning Sunshine" in my brain.)

Another theory has to do with the research done on the phenomenon known as an out-of-body experience (OBE). Those who have had a classic OBE, know it! An OBE is described as an event where the energy-body or etheric-body separates from the physical body for a brief time and then spontaneously returns. In the classic experience, the individual is very aware of being able to see the physical body from a vantage point outside the body. It is probably most often experienced as the result of surgery, anesthesia, traumatic injury, near death, a drug-induced state of consciousness or an accident. My first occurred when I was 13, and participating in a church discussion when I realized I was viewing the entire affair from a "shelf" high above the group. Others followed as the result of an explosion, and years later, thanks to a prescription painkiller.

One of the pioneers in research of this state of consciousness was Robert Monroe, a sound engineer who began having such experiences spontaneously in his middle years. As an engineer, he wanted to know how these events happened and whether he could exert any control over them. His groundbreaking research started in a spare room in his home and ultimately resulted in the creation of the world-renowned Monroe Institute in Faber, VA. In the process of researching what made "re-connecting" with the physical body or the host more difficult at times, he discovered that the presence of reflective surfaces in the room was the common denominator in all of these difficult re-entries. He theorized that the reflection in mirrors of multiple images of the host makes it hard to identify the real host, interfering with re-entry.

Whatever the cause, I've found that either moving the bed to a more private position or removing or covering the mirrors in the room can remedy many long-standing sleep problems. One of my sons began having difficulty sleeping after he moved his bed in front of double, mirrored doors. Since he resisted moving the bed, I hung posters on the mirrors and the sleep problem was solved. In other situations, sheer drapes covering the doors during sleep times will do the trick. They are easily opened during hours of use and add a sense of elegance to the room. One client had experienced insomnia for the entire twenty years she'd lived in her home. Since moving the bed was not an option, I suggested she hang sheer curtains to separate a mirrored dressing alcove from her bedroom. From the moment she hung the curtains, she no longer had trouble falling asleep or staying asleep. She called me later to confess that she thought it sounded like hocus-pocus, and was stunned that it worked so quickly and effectively.

Desks or workout equipment in bedrooms

Work-related equipment or furniture can also reduce the quality of sleep, because we never quite disconnect from the work associated with these pieces. Bedrooms should be about rest, sleep, and intimacy. I don't recommend the placement of studies off the bedroom unless the doors connecting these rooms can be totally closed off during sleep periods.

Artwork and accessories

Decorative accessories should be positive and uplifting and if photographs are used, they should be of happy people and events. For couples, there is a suggestion that pictures of children, grandchildren and friends can interfere with physical intimacy. After all, catching a glimpse of your two-year-old granddaughter is not particularly conducive to intimacy. Don't assume that your parents no longer care about intimacy just because they are aging. Studies and stories affirm that our need for physical intimacy continues to be an important part of life even though it may change in frequency or character.

Avoid hanging shelves or framed artwork over the head of the bed for obvious reasons. Shelving is particularly unsafe and gives the feeling that you always have "something hanging over your head!" Even if you are not aware of these feelings at a conscious level, they can interfere with sleep. One client complained of sleep problems since moving into her new home. Upon arrival I saw that her bed was in Position 5 (in front of the door) and had a decorative shelf hung about three feet above the headboard. We move the bed to the opposite wall (Position 1) and her sleeping problems were remedied.

The following comments have come from client letters I've received after rearranging the sleeping space according to these guidelines. They tell the story far better than I can.

> "I am reporting in progress. I rearranged my bedroom over the weekend. I took down the mirror. Got rid of the TV. Made certain there was nothing under the bed, etc. I slept better this week than I have in ages. I am not kidding. Thank you so much!!!!!"
>
> —Josie in Austin

"You asked me if I had trouble sleeping after entering my Master Bedroom. I said that I had always had trouble sleeping—both falling asleep—but especially staying asleep. You advised me to put a drape across the foot of my canopy bed. After you left I put a sheer drape up—to block the energy from the bathroom. I sleep like a baby that night—and every night since then. AMAZING!!! First time in at least 20 years!!!"

—Linda in West Virginia

Office or Study

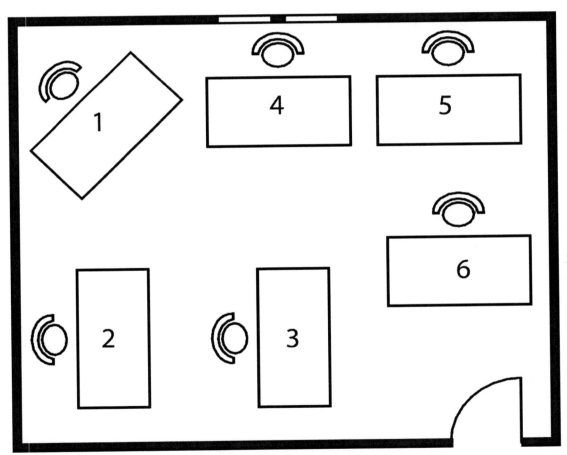

Diagram 2: Desk Placement

The rules-of-thumb for desk placement are as follows:

- Desks should face into the room and NOT face the wall;

- They should also have the largest view of the room;

- The user of the desk should have a view of the door.

An interesting thing happens when we push a desk against the wall so that we have no distant view. I hear comments like "I feel like I'm always running into a brick wall!" and "I feel there's no place to go in this job!" The other symptom is having no real view of the future.

An entirely different problem comes from sitting with your back exposed to the door. When choosing a seat in a café, nearly everyone I know will sit with his/her back to the wall. It's a natural protective instinct to want to know what's going on behind our backs. When we sit with back exposed, even in a safe place, we still tend wonder what's happening and that diverts part of our attention from the task at hand. Sitting with our back to the door results in reduced productivity, creativity and focus, and simultaneously increases stress and fatigue. A very successful attorney I worked with moved his office and no longer wanted to spend time there. He complained of fatigue, general malaise and lack of productivity. All the furniture in his office was the same as in his previous office, as were personnel. The only change was in the arrangement of the space: this arrangement had his back exposed when he sat at his computer work. A simple reconfiguration of the space solved the problem and simultaneously improved the comfort his clients felt when entering the room.

Computers

The issue of computers always comes up in these discussions, because people worry about all the cords. The cure for this is pretty straightforward and involves bundling the cords and using a plant behind the computer as camouflage. The plant can be silk or real and either way adds a sense of life force in the room. The important thing is to have a view of the room when working at the computer.

The Power Position

The name of this position says it all. Position 1 shown above in Diagram 2 has the largest view of the room and commands the space. Position 2 works well, but doesn't feel as commanding. I've experienced the shift that occurs when a desk is moved from facing the wall, back-exposed-placement to the "power position," and it is dramatic. A simple change in arrangement results in the feeling of greater control over life, a view of things to come and heightened organization. Clients using this position in both home and work spaces report positive shifts in work habits and that they feel more relaxed and confident. I've also seen both personal and business relationships dramatically improve as the result of this change.

Oddly, arrangements like this make the room feel larger and more functional, but represent a shift away from the more dated habit of lining all the furniture along the wall to leave a large open space in the middle. What we're after here is optimum function and aesthetics, not empty space in the middle. Positioning the desk so the door can be seen also makes it easier to communicate because of our growing dependence on visual cues. Individuals with hearing loss naturally tend to "tune-out" to the great frustration of those who live with them, and sitting with the back to the door only exacerbates that problem.

Position 4 could be good, were it not for the window behind the seat, which can have a reduced version of back-to-the-door. Positions 5 and 6 are too exposed except for short-term projects. We know that people seated facing the door suffer more interruptions and spend less time at the desk.

As with every room arrangement, the goal is to optimize and work within the constraints of the particular environment. If it is absolutely necessary to face the desk toward the wall, placing a mirror in a position so that if reflects the door is a possible "fix." That way, one can see what's going on behind by looking in the rear-view mirror.

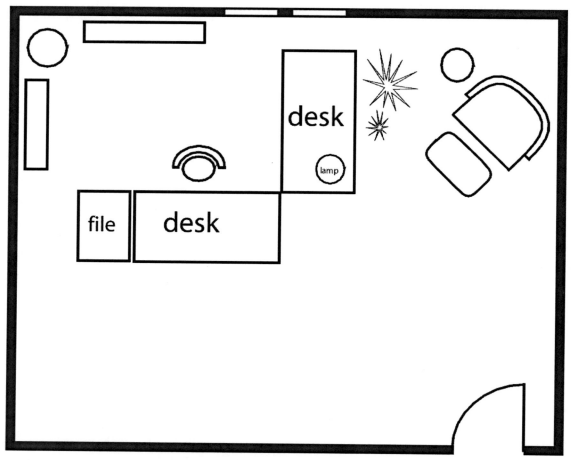

Diagram 3: Office Configuration

This shows one option for an ideal configuration for an office, whether at home or work. Either seating position at the desk allows a view of the door. The L-desk with bookcases behind offers an ideal, ergonomic workstation with easy access to both files and bookcases. The desk perpendicular to the window offers a view of the outside and the door, as well as communication with a guest sitting in the chair. Alternatively, the chair provides a comfortable reading station with its own lighting. Plants hide computer cables and add life-energy and comfort to the space.

Living Spaces

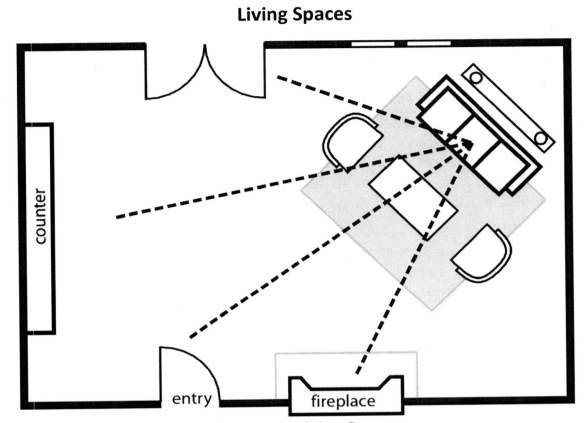

Diagram 4: Living Space

Family rooms or living rooms feel the most comfortable and function best when you can see all focal points from the primary seating. In the example shown in Diagram 4, there are four competing focal points—the kitchen bar (counter), double doors leading to the backyard, the fireplace and the entry door. The couch is positioned at an angle to the corner to be able to see all of these and the no-backs-to-the-door rule is satisfied because everyone can see the ENTRY door.

The entire arrangement is anchored by an area rug, and the table behind the couch accommodates two lamps, providing excellent reading light and atmosphere by warming the corner.

Notice that the furniture is arranged in a U-configuration that accomplishes two things:

- It embraces people as they come through the entry door with "open arms;"

- Pieces are positioned at right angles to each other to invite comfortable conversation.

All of the following configurations would technically work in that they all fit the space. None are quite as inviting as Diagram 4. Frequently there are complicating factors—more doors, built-in bookcases, too much furniture... In every case, it's a matter of finding the *optimum* arrangement, balancing use, mobility and special needs. Here's a portion of a letter written by Katie, a client in Austin who was stunned at the difference these arrangements made. I include it because Katie mentions the resistance many people feel to moving their furniture around.

"When Nancy arrived at my home, we began the process by looking at each room. I was surprised when Nancy asked if she could move some furniture around in my office. I didn't know that furniture moving was part of Feng Shui. After about 20 minutes of my explaining to her that none of her furniture moving ideas would work in my office, Nancy suggested we leave the office and go into the living room. In my living room, I also explained why the furniture needed to be where it was.

Then I started laughing and asked Nancy, 'Do you think there is any way I could be in resistance?' I thought I was open to this, but maybe I'm not. Help me out here!

Nancy said, 'Yes, you probably are in a little resistance, and that's okay, because that's pretty normal. Will you let me move a couple of things? If you don't like it, I'll move them back.' That was the beginning of the transformation of my home (and of my attitude!) The difference in the living room once she moved the furniture was so immense that I truly don't have the words to express it. I was so excited by the difference that I asked if we could go back to the office. We ended up moving furniture in three rooms and the difference is amazing."

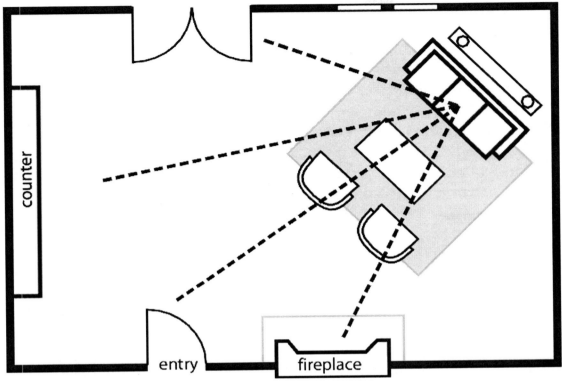

Diagram 5: Face-To-Face Seating

The face-to-face seating shown in Diagram 5 is much more formal and more adversarial in terms of communication. The chairs have these added disadvantages:

- Backs are turned to the kitchen, interfering with socializing;
- Backs are turned to the entry door;
- No view of the fireplace;
- Blocks the view of the fireplace from the couch.

A rough approximation of the above arrangement was in place in the home of Margie, a newly divorced client whose kids kept avoiding the living room and landed in her bedroom to visit and watch TV. We moved the furniture to roughly match Diagram 4, which also gave the kids a view of the front door. From that day forward, they never ended up in her bedroom again and loved hanging out in the newly designed living room. Here are her comments:

"My family was going through a terrible time in 1997... after a divorce and a wrenching move to a much smaller house. I was worried about children, finance and lawyers. I was so unhappy about moving and the house was not home. My family seemed to spend most of our time in our own rooms and ignored "family rooms." Nancy came over and went to work (moving furniture and accessories), and when she finished I was already less anxious and more positive about my new life. Later, another friend, Cindy, came over and was wowed by the difference! The house was warm and inviting to me now."

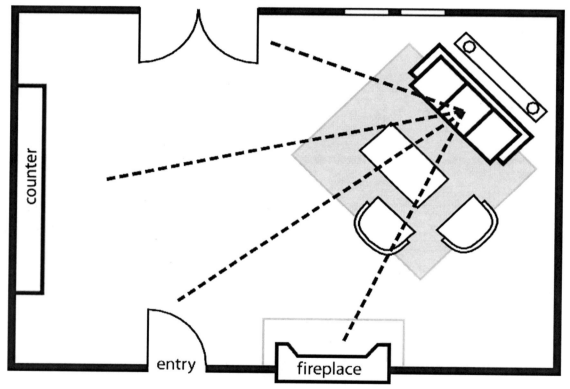

Diagram 6: Right Angle Placement of Chairs

The right-angle placement of the chairs in Diagram 6 has one chair with its back to the door and the fireplace, blocks the view of the fireplace from the couch and feels a little heavy on the right side.

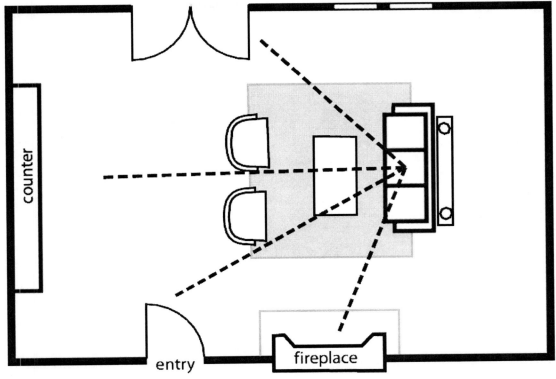

Diagram 7: Formal Arrangement

Seating in Diagram 7 feels more formal, and has the disadvantages of:

- Blocking people sitting in the chairs from any communication with the kitchen area;

- Two chairs with their backs to the entry door;

- Two chairs with no view out the double doors.

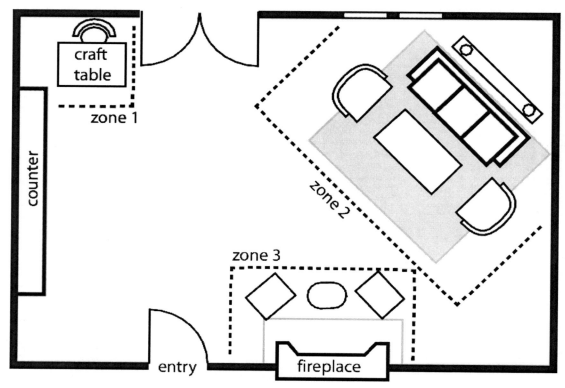

Diagram 8: Arranging Multiple Zones in a Large Room

Diagram 8 shows some possibilities for arranging multiple zones in a large room, increasing both comfort and functionality.

Other Environmental Factors

As important as spatial arrangements are the background factors of color, lighting, sound, and odor or fragrance in creating comfort, functionality and aesthetics. While each must be addressed as it is related to the personal tastes of the individual, we need to pay attention to a few underlying physiological factors such as sensory acuity and breathable air.

Lighting

The quality and type of lighting can influence mood, health, functionality, ability to understand speech, and communication. Overhead light, while functional, doesn't do much to create an ambience of comfort and warmth. Lamps and accessory lighting do more for creating an emotionally welcoming atmosphere.

Less than optimum lighting can contribute to a feeling of dis-ease and can interfere with doing the most basic tasks. As we age, some eye conditions interact with lighting to interfere with clear vision. One of those conditions is cataracts, which scatter light, reduce the amount of light reaching the retina and can make images blurry. Glare exacerbates the problem and also interferes with lip reading and therefore communication. Arrange seating according to the following guidelines:

- The listener is not facing directly into the glare.

- Eliminate glare bouncing off surfaces and coming from lamps as much as possible.

- Provide adequate task lighting for reading, hobbies and navigation.

- Provide dimmers where possible.

- Be sure lamp switches and twist knobs can be managed. Arthritis and weakened joints make it hard to turn lamps on and off. Therefore, consider touch lights and pull chains. Any metal lamp can be turned into a touch lamp with a device than inserts into the bulb receptacle. Lamps that turn on to the sound of hands clapping are also an option.

The AGS Foundation for Healthy Aging suggests that a 75-watt bulb placed two feet away is sufficient for reading. For those who have difficulty going from bright light to reduced light, transitional lighting is recommended. Using a small lamp or night light in bathrooms or interior rooms without any natural lighting will also help, especially moving from a night-darkened bedroom into a bathroom.

Color

Both hue and intensity of color have a physiological impact as well as psychological ramifications. While there are individual variations depending on personality, warm colors—those with a yellow base (yellows, reds, oranges)—are generally agreed to be associated with emotions ranging from feelings of warmth and comfort to feelings of anger and hostility.

Cool colors—those with a blue undertone, including blue, purple, and green, are generally associated with the emotions of calm, but can also elicit feelings of sadness or indifference.

It has been said that warmer colors, those with a yellow undertone, can raise the perceived temperature of a room, and cool colors lower the perceived temperature. While there is anecdotal evidence to support this, the research is not conclusive. Because elderly people often have poorer circulation and tend to be more stationary, being cold or having cold hands and/or feet is a common complaint. It's worth working with color to help ameliorate this problem.

In any case, great attention should be paid to your parent's personal preferences. Color choices are extremely individual and the same colors that make one person feel happy and centered can be downright nauseating to another. I've changed hotel rooms because I couldn't spend the night in a brown room, while clients have been quite content in a brown environment. I've also noticed that there seem to be "brown" people and "gray" people and each is profoundly unhappy living in the "other" color. Pay attention to your responses to color and do whatever you can to surround yourself with colors you really love and help your parents do the same.

Sound

Every aspect of sound plays a significant role in our ability to feel connected to the world in that it influences everything from our ability to hear warning noises to understanding what people are trying to say to us. Even low-level background noise can be irritating, and high intensity, low-frequency sound in the vibratory range (when it can be felt, more than heard) can cause fatigue, a feeling of dis-ease and a sense of foreboding. Higher frequency noises are especially irritating and at intense amplitudes can cause temporary and permanent sensory-neural (nerve damage) hearing loss. We know most of this, but it bears attention both when choosing a place to live and making the chosen spot more inviting and comfortable. In looking back, I realize my first foray into the power of sound to influence us came while writing a sixth grade essay on the role of music in emotion. I've played piano since second grade and this seemed like an easy paper to write. Now there is research to back up English playwright William Congreve's quotation "Music hath charm to soothe the savage breast." Yes, it does say breast, even though controversy still rages over whether he meant to say beast or breast. Since the quote came from the Latin "Musica delinit bestiam feram," it's possible he meant beast. Either way, it makes its point. The full quotation from *The Mourning Bride* (Congreve, 1697) is "Music hath charm to soothe the savage breast, to soften rocks or bend a mighty oak."

We know that the music of Mozart, for example, promotes healing, strategic problem solving and mathematical ability. (See *The Mozart Effect,* Campbell, 1997). In houses for sale, playing classical music in the background adds a touch of class to any property. In setting up a space for your Mom and Dad, see that music is available and that the sounds they are exposed to are comforting and calming. The sounds of a fountain can run the gamut from masking more disagreeable sounds like traffic noise, to making you want to run to the bathroom, if the trickling sound isn't "just right." White noise from running water, a dishwasher, or the air conditioner can interfere with speech comprehension because—as we will address in Chapter 13 on Special Needs—it masks the higher frequency consonant sounds, while leaving the lower frequency vowel sounds intact. The result is hearing, but not understanding.

Odor

Different fragrances or odors can cause us to feel cranky or soothed and can be related to air quality or just sensory preferences. A high quality air-purifier can reduce allergens and mold content as well as make the air smell fresher. Moldy environments cause sinus infections, upper-respiratory infections, headache, and obviously negatively impact health. Many people are allergic to perfumes, air fresheners, the out-gassing that results from many new paints, coatings, fabric dyes, carpet, and wallpaper paste. Be alert to changes in health soon after moving into a new home and remain open to the possibility that air quality may be the culprit. If the smells of strong cleansers such as Clorox, Lysol or pine oil are present, try less offensive alternatives. Medication odors and those resulting from incontinence can be reduced by using air-purifiers. Potpourri, sweet smelling candles and plug-ins may hurt more than they help. If you need a nice fresh fragrance, try a bowl of fresh lemons, a bunch of Rosemary or natural lavender.

Summary and Major Points

1. Prepare for movers and divesting of larger pieces of furniture by creating a plan of The Big Picture.

2. Arrange bedrooms for privacy and recuperative rest, using Diagram 1 as a reference.

3. Avoid clutter, desks, and workout equipment in the bedroom.

4. Artwork accessories, colors, sounds and texture should be supportive and uplifting.

5. Arrange offices and/or desk areas for productivity and safety, avoiding facing desks to the wall or seating the user's back the door

6. Arrange living spaces to invite the user with open arms; U-shaped and L-shaped arrangements are best, utilizing multiple focal points.

Suggested Activities

1. List the furniture you know you have a use and space for.

2. List those items you would like to take, but are optional in terms of use.

3. Think of ways you might use the optional items and incorporate them in a functional way that does double duty and might allow you to take them. For example:

- A loved drop leaf table than you no longer need as a dining room table could be placed behind a sofa to provide interest, dimension and a place for reading lamps.

- A favorite end table can be transformed into a bedside table.

- A needed file cabinet used for archived documents can double as an end table by having a circular top cut and covering all with a beautiful round table cloth.

- Baskets, instead of being purely decorative, can be serve as active storage in open shelving, a pantry, bathrooms, or for craft storage.

- An old dining room table can be given new life as a desk, display area for artwork, or family photos, an antique high-chair can make a beautiful plant stand in an otherwise dead corner; or an old quilt can be hung on a bare wall as artwork or make a visual headboard.

4. Using graph paper, sketch your rooms and experiment with furniture placement. If you like, cut furniture pieces to scale and try different pieces in alternative arrangements.

10

Unpacking, Settling in, The Little Pieces

Before Arriving

If at all possible, have the basic utilities and services (gas, electricity, water and telephone) turned on prior to the arrival of the van at the other end of the move. If you need computer access immediately, arrange for Internet connections at the same time. For those of you accustomed to moving, this may all be just too obvious. However, for folks who have been in the same house for the last forty years, and those who have always had a spouse take care of such things, the effort of getting accounts established can be daunting. In some cases, new accounts must be opened in person. When moving Mom I was dismayed to discover that account reps would not allow me to open the account FOR her on the telephone without HER speaking to them to communicate her permission for them to speak to me. Since the primary reason for my making the call in the first place was her hearing problem, it was ludicrous for them to have to have a conversation with her before they could converse with me. So, beware!

Van Arrival

By the time the van arrives, hopefully you've made at least some preliminary decisions about where furniture will be placed. If you don't, movers may make decisions that will be backbreaking and time-consuming later. Have the plan in hand on moving day and share it with your movers. Move in will be faster, the movers will love you for planning ahead and the biggest payoff is that when you start unpacking, you can unload directly into the pieces because they'll be in the right place to begin with.

If your parents are easily fatigued or overwhelmed, attempt to convince them to stay at a hotel or the home of a friend or relative on the day the truck arrives. As much as they may want to be present to supervise and have input, this can be self-defeating, exhausting for everyone and particularly frustrating for your elderly parent. There is no place to sit, rest, get comfortable or eat while the chaos is underway. It will help if you have gone over room arrangements ahead of time so they trust that you won't arrange their things without their input. Above all they *do not want to be managed!* If they know their wishes are being honored, they'll be much more likely to let you "manage the move." All of the detailed discussion, creative visualization and the pains you have taken to determine what matters most will pay off here, because they will already have had important input into this phase of the move. They don't have to be physically present during move-in to have their voice heard.

You might explain that you're taking care of that day as part of your "gift" to them, to be sure they are well rested and that some basics will be put into place by the time they get there. Moving is exhausting for anyone, but more so the older you get. If this is a long-distance move, you can get the movers to provide an estimated time of arrival so you have some latitude. Give yourself time to drive at a comfortable pace, get ensconced in lodging and get your parent(s) temporarily settled before the movers arrive. It may take older people days to recover before they are ready to help with the process, and the more you can have unpacked and in place, the better. When my mother moved from Lake Charles to San Marcos, one (extremely) good friend and I had her totally moved in and unpacked in two to three days. Later, another friend helped me hang the artwork. Mom arrived on scene after all the furniture was in place, clothes hung, and the bathroom and kitchen operational. That way, she was able to enjoy the process of deciding which books she wanted where and which artwork she wanted to see every day (living room and bedroom) and which she just wanted "around" (study and guest bathroom).

How much your folks can contribute depends on strength, endurance and pacing. Hiring a professional organizer can be very helpful, but be sure you interview the organizer at length about their history, training and philosophy before leaving them to work with your parents. Ask specifically if they have worked with the elderly and will communicate with them about their preferences. I've had to repair a lot of emotional damage inflicted by "helpers" who acted autonomously, discarded important papers or neglected to communicate with their clients. The role of the helper is to offer ideas where needed, but to listen closely to the preferences and needs of the client. The best system is designed to recognize and support the client's habits and natural tendencies, and make it work for them instead of against. A good system does not require the client to have to bend around it.

Further, clients with special needs will obviously require special attention. Determine whether your organizer has had training or experience in working with your particular need set, or spend some time being very specific about special requirements.

Where to Start?

Nutrition

Before you start unpacking, get some basic high quality snacks and drinking water on hand. Unpacking takes not only physical energy, but mental energy as well. Since the primary organ needed for unpacking, making organizational decisions and setting priorities is the brain and the brain is an electrical mechanism, water is essential to cognitive processing and *mood*. Hydration is essential to this process.

Furthermore, the brain consumes 30% of the body's calories. So feed it with protein, complex carbohydrates, and water. A good supply of Omega 3 fatty acids will help with processing and making decisions. You can take it in capsule form or get it in foods like cold-water fish, walnuts, ground flax seeds and whole grains. Daniel Amen, M.D., in his book, *Change Your Brain, Change Your Life* lists the best brain foods as:

Blueberries	Beans	Broccoli	Walnuts
Oranges	Salmon	Oats	Tea
Pumpkin	Tomatoes	Spinach	
Soy Beans	Yogurt	Turkey	

Clear as you go

Breaking down the boxes and bagging and packing materials one item at a time will help create space and give you a feeling a real progress. Whether you're putting the boxes at the curb, giving them away or taking them to recycling, they'll need to be flattened. If you can get started while the movers are bringing things in, many times the carrier will take the broken-down boxes and some of the packing material with them for future clients to use.

Which rooms first?

Conventional wisdom says to start with the kitchen and then the bedroom, but that assumes that cooking is a high priority. Certainly that's true with a family with kids that need to be fed on schedule and frequently, but priorities change...

- My first choice is the **bedroom**, because at the end of a stressful day, what we can't get anywhere but our own bedroom is a good night's sleep. And the older we get, the more critical it becomes and the longer takes to recover from a lost few hours. If your parent has resisted the invitation to remain off-site during the day, this room is a critical first step.

- You'll sleep better if you can locate enough towels and toiletries to be able to shower that night and get yourself comfortable. (Remember to pack those with the other essentials that are brought in the car).

- For anyone with health issues, locate **medications** and **health equipment** and put those in a safe place where they can be found quickly and they don't disappear in the ensuing chaos. Other medications and bathroom supplies can wait until later.

- If you're operating a business or are in daily contact with clients or family via the computer, your next priority might be the **computer.** For some of us (and I include myself in this category) being disconnected from cyberspace is tantamount to being stranded on an alien planet.

- Do the **kitchen** next, at least in terms of the basics. This is especially true if you're dealing with special dietary needs relating to blood sugar.

- **Area rugs** should be put down before heavy furniture to avoid having to get help moving the furniture later. Even if they have to be adjusted, they are out of the way and the place begins to feel like home faster.

After these basics, go for what will make you feel at home the fastest. **Lamps** are a high priority for me because overhead lighting alone does nothing to make a place feel homey. Remember, lamps are what create warmth and a sense of ambience.

You may have noticed by this time that I'm not just going for function here. After a few critical items like those listed above, function only goes so far. What will make your new digs feel like home the fastest is getting to the things that create that "sense of place" talked about in Chapter 2.

For me, it's the *artwork*. I need my pictures hung to feel like I live in a place, and if you've done your homework about furniture placement, you'll be ready to hang pictures within a couple of days. Really! As I mentioned before with Mom, it was only after her pictures were hung that the twinkle in her eye returned... For you, it may be getting your kitchen completely in order, for others it's the office or the art studio or the stereo system or the birdbath in the backyard. It's not the same for everyone. Use the discoveries you made at the end of Chapter 2 to guide you.

When arranging artwork, placement and grouping can create a feeling of warmth and balance, or feel disjointed and dated. In the Diagram 9 below, the wide, disorganized spacing of the five pieces feels dated, causes the eyes to jump around, and lacks focus.

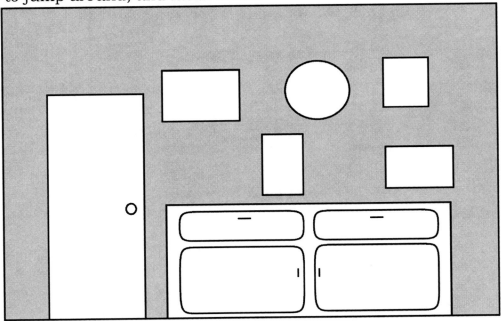

Diagram 9: Arranging Artwork Randomly

In the next diagram, individual pieces are hung in a tight group that feels cohesive and shows off the five pieces as a single group. It feels more organized, balanced and current.

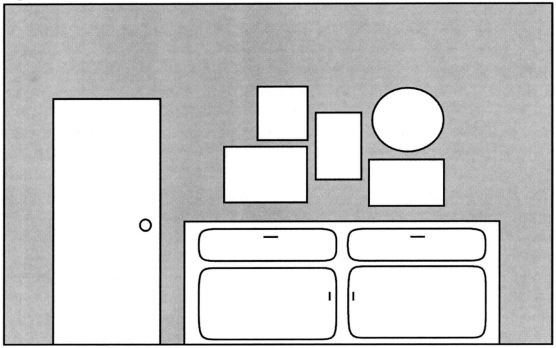

Diagram 10: Arranging Artwork in a Group

Creating Space

Regardless of the square footage of your parents' new place, everyone can benefit by taking advantage of vertical storage. The need to optimize space is especially evident in the pantry, bathroom and the garage, if there is one. Residents of several retirement communities complaining of the scarcity of functional storage have found these ideas useful and easy to implement. They can easily double or triple your usable space.

In General

- **Turntables** in the kitchen, pantry and bathrooms keep everything accessible. Double-decker versions have twice the usable area and they are available at nearly every discount store and certainly places like organizing specialty stores.

- **Stackable drawers** come in a zillion different shapes, materials, colors and dimensions. They can help organize cosmetics, medications by type, office supplies, craft materials, tools—nearly everything. Use them in the office closet to store supplies, in the clothes closet to make extra room for things that look messy folded on a shelf, or anywhere else you have empty vertical space. Units that fit between washer and dryer can hold tools, light bulbs or laundry supplies. Drawers are superior to stacking boxes because they avoid the requirement of lifting boxes to get to items on the bottom. We're seldom in the mood to restack boxes after we've found what we're looking for, leaving a trail of disarray.

- **Pegboard** hung in the garage, pantry or closet can house tools, belts and hats to keep them handy, freeing up valuable shelf or drawer space.

- **Industrial racks** or grids can be used anywhere for a clean, efficient method of hanging anything that can fit on a peg. Many have the means of creating hanging bins for small hobby supplies, utensils, or tools.

- **Double rods** (or the equivalent) are useful in the closet for shirts and pants.

- **Stacking shoe bins** get shoes out of piles on the floor and work better than racks.

- **Ziplock® bags** keep small items together and help organize drawers.

- **Functional art:** baskets and pottery usually used just for decoration can do double duty to attractively store items and reduce visual clutter.

- **Stackable vinyl racks** such as those put together with tubular supports are easy to assemble, inexpensive and versatile for use in the garage, storage or deep closets. When not in use they can be bundled into cubes. Built-in adjustable shelving is also an option if you have the time and resources.

Ideas for vertical storage

- Pegboards or hooks for tools;
- Floor to ceiling utility shelves;
- Wall or ceiling mounted racks for bikes, fishing gear and sports equipment;
- Loft-like shelving around the periphery for lightweight, out of season or seldom used items;
- Stackable plastic sorting bins or drawers for smaller items.

Other bathroom tips

- Vertical bins with drawers: store like items together;
- Custom drawer dividers;
- Attractive baskets or pottery to group items that remain in view;
- Labels on drawers or shelves (you don't need to be obvious);
- **Accessible** laundry hamper.

Setting Up Each Room—Getting Specific

The following guidelines offer a framework for arranging and setting up each room in the house. Using this framework will result in a space that is not only more comfortable and inviting, but functional in that it optimizes privacy, physiological ease, ergonomic factors, and psychological well-being.

Living/family Rooms

- Locate a natural focal point (not necessarily the television);
- Face furniture to accommodate the outside view (if pleasant), or fireplace, or both;
- U-shape arrangements are more conversational and inviting;
- Pay attention to glare, conversational distance and maneuvering room;

- Arrange the "U" so that it welcomes with "open arms" when entering the room;

- AVOID: couch-back-to-the-entry-door;

- Move TV cable nearer to the natural focal point so the arrangement takes in everything relevant;

- Use lamps for atmosphere. They are softer and more welcoming;

- Tie the arrangement together with an area rug if available;

- Round the corners with plants and/or lighting for warmth and atmosphere;

- Task lighting should be within each reach and accommodate dexterity requirements (avoid hard to turn switches in favor of toggle switches, pull chains or tap lighting);

- If the room is large, create zones for smaller conversational groups, games or special projects.

Bedroom

- Arrange the bed for privacy;

- Adjust bed height for safe entry and exit;

- Provide a place to sit for reading, or putting on clothing;

- Lamp by the chair;

- Use a headboard to provide a sense of permanence and safety;

- Provide bedside tables with a drawer and room for telephone, glasses, medications, books, water glass, lamp;

- Create rounded edges on furniture in traffic corridor if falling is an issue;

- Nothing should be stored under the bed, to allow for good airflow and avoid dust accumulation;

- Remove work desks/computers;

- Choose restful or cheerful art work;

- "Peaceful and private" are the key words.

Offices

- Place the desk in the command position;
- Face the desk to view the room: NOT facing wall;
- The desk seat should not be "back to door;"
- Arranging the work area in "L" or "U" position is best;
- Active files should be within each reach and visible if necessary;
- Position the computer to allow view of the room while working;
- Bundle and hide equipment cables for safety and aesthetics;
- When needed, add book cases for vertical storage;
- Store and file like with like;
- Label files and folders with a Label Maker to allow easy reading and access;
- Use task lighting on desk;
- Provide a glare screen for computer if required.

Bath

- Use non-slip rugs for warmth, safety and acoustics;
- Install grab rails in shower and tub;
- A small lamp or nightlight adds safety and convenience;
- Baskets or attractive containers can be used for toiletries;
- Non-slip bath or shower mats improve safety;
- Maximize vertical storage in cabinets;
- A turntable under the sink offers easy access to supplies.

Garage

- Create vertical storage using shelves to accommodate large storage boxes;
- Pegboard is useful for flat tools, hoses, garden rakes;

- Shelves or small table by the door provide storage for things going out;
- Paint the walls with a light color, high gloss paint for easy cleaning and light reflection;
- Add task lighting for fix-it projects;
- Reduce or eliminate piles of debris, clutter, and tools;
- Room for cars is a must!

Summary and Major Points

1. Before arriving, have basic utilities, (including computer access if desired) turned on.

2. If possible, arrange for your parent to stay with a friend or hotel on move-in day. Prior discussion of placement will help put them at ease.

3. Support yourself and your parent during the process by packing nutritious snacks, ample water, and taking at least at a 10 minute break each hour.

4. Put rugs down first to avoid having to move furniture later to lay them.

5. Break down boxes and clear packing materials as you go.

6. Determine which rooms or items (bedroom, medications, kitchen, etc.) are the most critical for your parents' comfort and start creating order there.

7. After the essentials are under control, take time to feed the soul by putting some of their treasures in place so they begin emotionally connecting to the space.

8. Much additional storage can be created by maximizing on vertical storage with shelves, drawers, pegboard and double hanging racks in the closet.

9. After major pieces are in place, use the detailed guidelines and your parents' input to fill in the blanks.

Suggested Activities

1. List the things you will want immediate access to. Possibilities include medications, nightclothes, towel and washcloth, toiletries, pillow, bed linen. Start a suitcase that you can add to as you think of things.

2. Organize your unpacking box and put it in your car to take with you. Include the following:
   - Box cutters;
   - Floor plans;
   - Snacks;
   - Water;
   - Large plastic garbage bags;
   - Picture hangers;
   - Hammer;
   - Pliers;
   - Flash light;
   - Furniture sliders.

11

Heart Strings

The furniture is arranged, toothbrush in place, phone hooked up and already ringing with pesky solicitations, groceries are in and cable-TV hooked up. You're finished, right? Not really... whether you're moving Mom and Dad, or yourself, mind and spirit become engaged only as you make connections.

Road Maps and Transportation

Having just more or less completed the physical process of moving Mom into her bright and airy new place, I was poignantly reminded that even though she had physically moved in, she was emotionally adrift. I know that may seem obvious, but it's really easy to trick ourselves into thinking that once everything is put away and they're physically safe and sound, our job is done, especially if we've taken time away from husband, kids and job. The act of moving is such a Herculean task, we tend to forget that the real measure of success depends on connecting to community, knowing your way around and feeling like you can get groceries, medications, and have your hair done without getting lost, depending on someone else, or doing without.

Mom, an unusually independent woman, had enjoyed a career, taken care of her yard, traveled, and in her 70s had done strenuous volunteer work that most of us wouldn't tackle in our thirties. She was brought to a standstill with the newest challenge of things as basic as getting a loaf of bread, buying stamps, or having a prescription refilled in a new city half the size of the one she'd just left. The move she accomplished to a new city at the age of 76 is far more difficult when repeated 10 years later. The four-way stop between her complex and the grocery store may as well be a parachute jump for the fear it arouses; she worries whether she'll be able to get to the pharmacy two blocks down the street because there's a left turn across four lanes of traffic. She wonders if her life will simplify with this move as anticipated, or has she made the move to the outer reaches of hell? I worry about that too... She ranks the loss of freedom that has resulted from this challenge as the single most difficult aspect of the move.

This dilemma isn't unique to the elderly. When I moved to West Virginia, there were all these little rural routes to the homes where I was to consult. If I took a wrong turn (and I did frequently), I could spend an hour finding my way out of the woods. Shepherdstown is a tiny little town about 60 miles Northwest of D.C., and driving 30 minutes in almost any direction could place you in any of three different states. This was a new experience coming from Texas, where it can take an entire day to cross a state line. In stopping to ask directions, sometimes I didn't even know what state I was in—other than in a state of frenzy. Although I soon discovered online maps, those would periodically drop me off in bizarre locations miles from my destination. Such events can be seen as an adventure at some stages of life, but as vision, attention and reflexes change for older adults, so does the ability to search for landmarks to find a new address, turning adventure into a nightmare.

Feeling lost—in more ways than one—undermines self-esteem, increases overall stress and fatigue and... it's dangerous. Statistics from the American Association of Motor Vehicle Administrators show that a 75-year-old driver is three times more likely to die in a car crash than a 23-year-old. The same parents, who may have been able to drive in their hometown or neighborhood, may become a hazard in an unfamiliar city and it may take some time to determine what they can manage.

As soon as possible, if driving is an option for your parents, you can speed up their adjustment by finding safe routes and practice driving those routes (with you as passenger) to basic amenities, which might include:

- Grocery store
- Pharmacy
- Library
- Church
- Family
- Friends
- Post office
- Discount store
- Elderly or disability friendly restaurants, theaters, etc

Ever noticed that most restaurants play fairly loud music that exacerbates the already deafening noise of clinking plates and forks and people talking? For the wearer of a hearing aid, this is impossible, because hearing aids amplify the background noise too. Naturally, there are places you will steer clear of, because they're designed for a different culture (teenagers, fast food, no conversation meals, etc.). I recently had an experience with a chain (Johnny Corrino's—just to be sure they get credit for their generous spirit and willingness to really serve the customer). I went ahead to reconnoiter the place, knowing it would be a no-go if loud music was the first thing heard. They willingly turned the music down and happily seated us in an area away from kitchen noise and high traffic patterns. This is rare, in my experience, and as a result we've been back many times. Each time, even though the wait-staff varied, we received the same accommodating treatment. In the same vein, some theaters offer assisted-listening devices.

Mobility challenges are also worth mentioning, because long before the need for a walker or a cane arises, there may be problems with picking the feet up high enough to step onto a curb. Diminishing vision can result in reduced depth perception, making it hard to distinguish a step up or down. Offer help or look for places with a ramp. Cataracts create problems with glare and being seated facing the window or bright light. Limited peripheral vision can create safety risks and a general lack of awareness of what's going on outside a limited field of vision. These and other challenges will be discussed in further detail as they relate to setting up the home environment.

Your parents' particular needs will vary. Whatever they are, a little time spent locating accommodating places will make entertainment forays so much nicer for all involved. The patterns we establish during the first few weeks after the move are important in defining later expectations and feelings of dependency or autonomy. The sooner we can offer solutions, make introductions, and establish new connections, the faster the adjustment. A dramatic move, such as that faced by our parents to a new city later in life, shares some of the characteristics of other traumatic events. My training as a Victim Services Counselor stressed the importance of offering caring and constructive support within the first few hours after an event, when people were more receptive. While you don't need to bombard them with new ideas on the heels of moving in, it is a good idea to start within the first few days or week.

After you've discovered a few new routes, ride as a passenger while your parent drives the route a few times, then create easy to read maps or typed directions (depending on the learning style of the user) and put them into a loose leaf binder with transparent sleeves. Leave them in the car for handy reference. If you're good at auditory processing, a navigation device that calls out the directions might help, but that requires being tuned in all the time, having excellent hearing, and not listening to the radio! It's not my cup of tea, but it works well for some people.

If you're helping parents adjust to a new place and find yourself constantly feeling responsible for getting them to locations that they were able to handle automatically in their old town, you may all worry that this present exhaustion is permanent; that their negativity over the place is there to stay and that you've all made an egregious error in moving. And as difficult as it is for us to adapt to having our parents newly dependent, it's even harder for them, emotionally.

Parents dislike having to ask their kids for help, so their "asking" may come disguised as:

- Complaining about not having something;

- Inviting you for dinner and—by the way—could we stop by Wal-Mart on the way?

- Dropping hints.

Sometimes it's hard to tell when we're being asked to "fix" something or asked to listen. I have a tendency to think I need to make it all better, but how many times have we been furious at our partner when we've just been venting and they jump in and try to tell us how to fix it—or they try to fix it for us? When in doubt, ask! A simple, "Would you like some help or do you just need someone to listen?" works wonders to take the edge off wondering, and exacerbating the problem by jumping in where you're not really needed. Another way to preserve your sanity, and theirs, is to get busy and find other forms of transportation, some of which have special rates or services for the elderly or disabled:

- On-Demand Public Transportation (e.g. CARTS);

- Taxi services;

- Elder Care;

- Agency on Aging volunteers;

- A neighbor;

- Church organizations.

Traveling in Fez, an ancient walled city in Morocco, I discovered a wonderful tradition offered to the elderly or homebound members of the community. All bread was taken to the local ovens for baking on a wooden board, to be picked up later in the day. Those who couldn't make it to the bakery simply left their dough by the door, knowing that someone would take it in for them. The baker knew which loaf belonged to whom based on the board it was on, and without any real planning, someone would see that the bread made it back to its maker. We can learn from such a system of caretaking and offer to help pick up groceries, medications and stamps for others as we go about our own errands. When we can do something as an act of generosity and blend it into our own routine, it can change it from being a "chore" to a gift. Small gestures such as these help us feel both cared for and caring.

And although we may not be able to provide fresh bread pickup and delivery, there are businesses that offer a home visit, provide transportation or delivery free or for a nominal charge. We located a pharmacy that delivers, a car repair shop that offers transportation both ways, an insurance agent to go to her home to make the necessary changes, and a taxi service accustomed to dealing with the particular needs of elderly clients. All of these were outside the more public services such as on-demand public transportation and mass-transit.

Birds of a Feather Flock Together... Finding Friends

Beyond the physical connections are the more important *emotional ones*: friends, and groups who share common interests and philosophies. Without those, YOU are the only connection and that portends trouble for both of you. Identities are compromised, dependencies become entrenched, and tensions escalate. No good can come of that.

Yes, it's up to them to some degree to ferret out those new friendships and associations, but it's not always easy in a new community—especially as you age. It takes a while to learn what's available. Everything you do within the first two weeks will pay off in spades later. Again, from the Victim Services example, left to their own resources, with no support or that which came too late, victims remained victims. I believe the same tendency applies to this trauma—and moving *is* a trauma.

Here's a partial list of things you can do to shorten the adjustment period and make everyone's life happier. Naturally, the degree to which help is needed depends on your parent's mobility, attitude, personality and interests, as well as what's available in their new community.

- **Libraries** are obviously a source for free reading material and computer access, but additionally they are a great resource to discover free classes, community events, clubs and organizations. It's a way to while away some hours, get a change of scenery and meet like-minded others. Volunteers are a valuable resource for smaller libraries that need help with cataloging, book sales, and behind the scenes support.

- **Churches/ synagogues** offer numerous programs and opportunities for learning, volunteer work and connecting with those who share a spiritual or religious outlook. Transportation is frequently available as part of the church's outreach.

- **Local theater** productions always need people to help with props, box-office, and other levels of volunteering, sometimes offering a comp-night in exchange for work.

- **Nature clubs** such as the Sierra Club and local versions offer an excellent opportunity for public service and social connections. Smaller communities have volunteer beautifications and culture groups offering community service in combination with day trips, lectures and teaching.

- **Charity thrift shops** operate almost entirely on the good will of volunteers, from organizing intake to front desk, depending on skills and the degree of public interface desired.

- **Public museums** offer those knowledgeable in history, art, and numerous specialty topics an avenue for sharing their knowledge with others while getting some of their public service and social needs met.

- **Literacy programs** offer teaching opportunities and the opportunity to work with those less fortunate.

- **Agencies on Aging** offer numerous services from support and transportation to information on state and federal services.

- **Bird watching** enthusiasts can find out about new haunts and group outings through the local Audubon Society. Trips are typically available for all levels of mobility and interests.

- **Informal classes** at colleges, public school districts and universities offer inexpensive venues for learning everything from how to get a book published to the latest dance steps and Feng Shui

- **Newcomers' groups** are alive and well in most communities and can be located via the Chamber of Commerce, local churches or a computer search. Sometimes these are so popular that people form lifelong friendships.

- **Elder Day Care** is a great resource for those with elderly parents at home who need an outside source of activities.

- **Elder Hostel** provides a nearly limitless list of possibilities for travel and education uniquely suited to a wide range of travel styles, finances and interests for elders. Resources and friends for travel, lodging and extended friendships last far beyond just the immediate trip.

- **Cooking classes** at your local Whole Foods or culinary school can offer both fun and a new base of friends who might like to form a dinner group.

Changes

If your move is out-of-state, you will also need to change:

- Medical prescriptions;
- Health care providers;

- Insurance policies;

- Vehicle registration (with or without having the title moved to another state);

- Driver's license;

- Voter registration.

Just for Fun

Doing things together that are NOT just need-based is a way of protecting your relationship against your feeling resentful over everything being a chore. Otherwise, this will feel like a relationship based on caretaking and not time spent with someone you love. One of the common complaints of adult children caring for parents has to do with arriving on scene to take them somewhere and being greeted with "While you're here..." Anticipate that some of this will happen because your folks really DO need some help with items and will save these up until you're coming over for some other reason. The danger that I see with this is that there is such a thing as "learned helplessness." They are perfectly capable of doing some things for themselves, but it's just easier to ask and then it becomes a habit.

Living in the same town as my grown son for the first time in seven years, I've noticed this tendency in myself—and it's not pretty. My relationship with my mother has been a useful mirror with which to examine my own relationship with my son. Living alone, I periodically come up against something I can't do myself—lift a heavy planter from my trunk, re-hang a cabinet door, dig a hole to bury the cat. These are all very real needs and I do need help, but recognizing my own response over the "while you're here" syndrome, I'm careful to seek help elsewhere when possible. When not, I will let him know I need some help when it's convenient for him and not load family dinners or impromptu visits with a list of chores.

I've discovered that one way to avoid this is to plan outings that are "just for fun" and have no work associated with them. That way the experience is "pure," and we can still enjoy each other as adults going out for a little adventure.

Don't be afraid to ask the question, "What would make your life here happier, easier, and more satisfying?" Sometimes in our effort to answer these questions without ever *asking,* we make ourselves crazy by second-guessing and making assumptions. Remember, some complaining is just *that*—and does not require a solution, just a willing ear. Simply moving in with our version of a solution can take away autonomy, dignity and the willingness to remain self-reliant to the greatest degree possible. **Asking** maintains the adult-to-adult relationship, shows concern without intrusiveness and shows that you really *are* listening.

Don't defend yourself or take the answers personally. This is not about you. It's very seductive to blame yourself or the other person in certain situations. One of these is when a family member is in need of help. You can assume you did something wrong, or are not doing enough, even if the other person doesn't think so. None of these responses are necessarily true, but they are all natural. Among the absolutely natural responses to taking care of a parent are:

- Guilt;
- Love;
- Anger;
- Pity;
- Resentment;
- Impatience;
- Blame;
- Self-recrimination;
- Feeling like a victim.

Summary and Major Points

1. After getting our parents physically settled, the next priority is to help them make connections and become autonomous.

2. One way to help with the settling-in process is to assist with finding routes to stores, physicians and friends, or helping them to locate alternative transportation. Possibilities are:

- On-Demand Public Transportation (e.g. CARTS);
- Taxi services;
- Elder Care;
- Agency on Aging;
- Neighbors;
- Church organizations.

3. A parent's becoming dependent on their adult children is emotionally difficult for both parties.

4. Establishing new connections within the first few weeks speeds up their adjustment and satisfaction with the move.

5. Seek out local volunteer opportunities or social organizations with interests or values similar to your parents', and determine how to help them connect. Some possibilities are:

- Libraries;
- Churches;
- Local theater;
- Nature clubs;
- Charity shops;
- Literacy programs;
- Public museums;

- Agencies on Aging;
- Bird watching clubs;
- Informal classes;
- Elder Day Care;
- Newcomers' clubs;
- Elder Hostels;
- Cooking classes.

6. Relocating out-of-state will require changing critical documents, including medical prescriptions, health care providers, insurance, registration, driver's license and voter registration.

7. Planning some activities that are just for fun, will balance the "caretaker" aspects of the relationship.

8. Ask your parent what would make their lives easier and more pleasant, instead of guessing.

9. Avoid defending yourself and don't assume you need to "fix" everything.

Suggested Activities

1. Talk with your parents and make a list of the places they most need to be able to visit.

2. Determine how that will happen: driving, public transportation, a bus arranged by their retirement complex, hired driver, etc. Make a list of phone numbers and leave it by the phone.

3. Make a loose-leaf folder with directions to routine or essential locations. The font size should be large enough to read comfortably from the driver's seat.

4. Talk with your parents about the type of activities or organizations they might enjoy and the best ways to facilitate the connections.

12

Little Rituals Make Us Feel At Home

Life is filled with little rituals. We wake up, stumble in to start the coffee, turn on the computer, click on e-mail, and go pour the coffee, come back and see what mail has popped up… At least that's *my* morning ritual. It's what gets me connected in the morning and if I'm without it—or without the crème that goes in the coffee, or have to use Splenda® instead of sugar, it throws me off. Not so much that I become a serial killer, but off nevertheless. A client of mine writes page after page in her journal before she gets out of bed and starts her more public day.

When I move into a new home, I have to put my mark on it as soon as possible. In addition to finding a place for all my coffee paraphernalia, this consists of hanging artwork. It's food for my soul. I'm compulsive about this and will decorate my walls before I get the rest of the kitchen stocked. After all, I can eat out, but I can't get my "soul-food" anywhere else. Another client knows she's found home when she's prepared a meal in her new kitchen.

It's the little rituals of life that make us feel at home, even away from home. They provide continuity in a changing world and performing them holds the mind in focus, slows its whirring and turns down the background noise. Do you take certain things with you when you travel? I'm not talking about your "rabbit's foot," although it could be that. Do you take a picture of your family and put it on the dresser before you fully settle in, perhaps a treasure from your child or your love to keep by the bed? Maybe you light a candle in the evenings and sit with a glass of wine, or read a few chapters before turning off the light.

Every religion, sorority, fraternity, club and sports team has its rituals. As in the bedtime stories we tell our children, rituals offer comfort, and serve a deeper purpose of connecting us to a larger context that identifies our relationship with the world and others. Ritual is the way we have of taking a hope or a desire into our hearts and performing a physical action to cement our commitment to a dream, a group or a belief. We take an oath, say a prayer, and wear a graduation robe or team colors to honor our intention.

Recognizing your personal rituals and making arrangements to honor them or put them in place quickly at your new home will make it *feel like home* sooner—while the motions offer comfort in the doing. Things as simple as having your own coffee brewed just the way you like it your first morning act as a bridge connecting your old life to the new one. (I grew up in Louisiana; we're big on our coffee rituals. In fact, my best memories of childhood all involve coffee!) In south Louisiana, you're actually weaned off milk onto milk-coffee as soon as you can hold a cup. First it's warm milk with sugar and just enough coffee to color the milk. As you get older, it's more coffee, less milk.

After high school graduation, my folks and I took a driving trip into central Mexico. On those long, desolate stretches we would find a puddle of shade under a tree and stop at about 10:00 in the morning and again in mid-afternoon. With a can of Sterno® and our travel coffeepot we made a strong pot of brew, laughed, shared our versions of experiences on the trip and honored generations before us—having coffee on the trail. It was continuity and social ritual. All things were christened with a cup of coffee.

What rituals do your parents hold dear? Mom's first ritual was to feed the birds she hoped to draw into her new life. Some clients need the TV hooked up to be able to stay in sync with a favorite TV show, others want the internet, in order to stay connected to their grandkids. Observing mid-afternoon tea during the move-in helps others.

One client owned puppies that were like her children. Immediately upon moving in, she set up the bedroom with ramps and pallets so her small companions could get on her bed where they would feel safe. Everyone has his or her own way to stay connected and maintain continuity. You will be able to find your own, but many rituals are so deeply woven into the fabric of our lives that a generation not given to introspection and self-analysis may be pressed to verbalize on them. So observe your Mom and Dad, see how they start and end their day, what activities they hold dear and which friendships they will feel bereft without. Take measures to see that those are in place or continued in some way to ease their stress and loneliness. Even contentious relationships can be missed when wrenched away.

Rituals to Provide Closure

Just as there are rituals that help welcome us to a new place, others help us leave one home and embrace another. Our ability to fully release the old place can make a difference in how fast it sells and how quickly we fully inhabit the new one.

This business of moving on is terribly personal. Our parents' generation was not as open about feelings, so may be uncomfortable about any planned ceremony. Still, the act of walking through the house, privately offering a prayer of gratitude for its shelter, might be all the ritual needed. It might also be too painful, so it shouldn't be forced.

When I moved from my home in Austin before heading "up north" as I called it, my house simply would not sell until I did some "releasing." As I've already mentioned, it's common knowledge in the real estate market that houses don't sell quickly if the owners are grieving over leaving. They're also slow to move when they are being vacated as the result of divorce, death in the family, financial distress or serious illness. Potential buyers sense something about the house at the front door and will come up will all manner of reasons why a "perfect house" that meets al their criteria "just won't work."

In the case of leaving Austin, I'd already purchased the house in Shepherdstown and was having it remodeled. My Austin home was beautiful, meticulously presented, priced right, in the right location—but would not sell. People came in, loved it, and commented on how calm and comfortable it felt, but a few mentioned that they "couldn't see their family living there," a common statement when there is so much "personal presence" or emotion anchoring the property. I didn't realize how deeply conflicted I was about leaving until I went to Costa Rica with friends for a "girls' week" at a beautiful home on a peninsula overlooking the Pacific Ocean. All of us were into spiritual things, so we each chose a ritual to help us with something we were working on. Mine of course had to do with selling my house, because the double payments were draining my reserves at a terrifying rate. Even though I'd chosen this move out of Texas, I was beginning to suspect that part of me really didn't want to leave. As an aging sailor, I designed a ritual to pull up my anchor from Austin. As a symbolic act, I made a little foil anchor, stuck it into some rocks representing Austin and pulled it out. Feeling more than a little silly as I did this, I was stunned when I exploded into tears. I really just couldn't bear to leave and this ritual brought it all to the surface where I could work with it.

Shortly thereafter, I moved my family pictures off the fireplace mantel and that opened another floodgate. That's when I realized this was really about my guilt over leaving the place the boys had always known as home. Never mind that *they* had already left; I felt in my heart it would still feel like home if "Mom" was there. One was in the Navy and the other pursuing his dream in California. Both gave their blessings. But I felt that if I left, I was moving their home and uprooting them. After it all came to the surface, courtesy of these rituals, the house sold in a week.

The point of my sharing this is to let you know how powerful our subconscious attachments are and how powerful rituals are in helping us move through loss and into new stages. Use them! Create your own! If you're helping a parent close up the family home, YOU may be the one who needs the ritual to help you both.

As you leave your old home, there are wonderful ceremonies you can do to bless its service to you and open it to its new owners or guardians. These help your leaving and bless it for those who come after you. I will offer them at the end of the chapter.

Starting with a Clean Canvas

Just as an artist wouldn't paint over another painting without cleaning the canvas, it's a good idea to energetically clean and bless your new house before or soon after you move in. Remember those old feelings that can be sensed in a house for sale? The home you're moving into also has some of the imprint of the previous owners (or even the construction crew). In Feng Shui, it's called Predecessor Energy. The previous occupants have left their imprint on the space your parents have just moved into, and it can influence how they adapt to life in that space. I'm not referring to hauntings, although I've cleared many a spirit. I really am just referring to the "vibes" that remain in a property after it's been vacated. Remember the Quantum Physics discovery that everything is vibrating? It turns out we weren't that far off in the 60s when we sang about "good vibrations."

I've heard of many properties that seem to have a history to them where the same types of events repeat over and over again. The good news is that the cycle can be broken by a simple act of intention. Intention used in conjunction with ritual is extremely powerful and I've learned to clear every house before or shortly after moving in. It's a routine part of my Feng Shui practice and there have been very interesting results.

Remember the house that wouldn't sell? That house was purchased at the end of a long central Texas summer—100 degree plus temperatures for a month, and I'd seen more houses than I could remember. I walked into this very cool, calm-feeling house and instantly thought, "Ah, this is what I need." I felt I could just sit right down and relax—take a little nap. It had been freshly painted a neutral off-white, had lovely D'Hannis tile floors, plantation shutters and a floor plan that worked. I made an offer and we closed and I moved in, in record time. Almost immediately after, I realized I was falling asleep the instant I sat down. "Hmmm, must be de-stressing after the divorce, law suit with the ex, hot summer, move, etc." After a while, I began to wonder about other things. I looked at the furniture arrangement again, colors, etc. I noticed the off-white had a lot of grey pigment in it and that is known to put people to sleep. I repainted it a nice soft white with a touch of yellow—it felt like liquid sunlight. That helped a bit, but when the boys mentioned that they were both sleeping too much and couldn't stay awake once they got home, I had to look deeper. What could this be?

Turns out, the previous and only owner was an anesthesiologist! Talk about leaving her energy behind—she was still doing a great job of putting people to sleep! I did another very thorough clearing and blessing of the space and the sleep issue disappeared.

Do your best to get a little history of the place before you move in, and then do your own clearing and blessing or hire a professional to do it for you. Feng Shui Consultants do this as a matter of course, but there are Native Americans who offer a ceremony, usually with sage, and others.

Housewarmings and Blessings

The ritual of inviting old friends and new neighbors over when you move into a new house seems a lost art. Believed to have originated with taking over hot coals to warm the new house, it became a way for young couples to start their life in a new home, with friends and relatives bringing gifts and food to warm both hearth and heart. In China it included bringing over a jar or rice to provide not only food, but the prospect of abundance. Today, rice is still used in many Feng Shui blessings. With people starting their independent lives much earlier as kids go off to school, this ritual isn't as much a part of the landscape as it used to be. Just because you don't need people to bring gifts is no reason not to invite them over. Simply announce that their company is the gift and have a welcome party. If your parent is new to your community, putting faces to the names of friends they've heard you talk about completes the circle. Both sides benefit from this sharing and your parent feels less adrift.

Most retirement communities have a Welcome Day to invite new residents into the fold. If not, you might help put something together for your parents once they've moved in. Since older folks may be embarrassed to have people see their place until everything is in place, you might move the party to the community room. Everyone likes free food and a reason to get out of the apartment once in a while, so don't worry about no one showing up!

Daily Rituals

Nothing will help put down roots faster than getting some of your *daily* rituals in place. Sometimes we don't even realize something is a ritual or discover how important an activity was until our routine has been disrupted. Only you will know what these are but you might recognize one in the list below.

- **Having breakfast at your favorite place** means you may need to find a *new* favorite place. You now have permission to start exploring!

- **Going for a morning walk** will help you work the kinks out after unpacking boxes, and walking in your neighborhood is a perfect way to meet your neighbors. Check out the local walking trails with the Chamber or naturalist group. Losing your walking route can have far-reaching consequences because it is directly or obliquely related to social life, sense of place, immunity, weight maintenance and body chemistry.

- **Taking Fido to the dog park** is a sure way to meet people who share at least one of your interests. It also keeps Fido happy and exercised. Our pet's wellbeing can be seriously disrupted by a move as well, and dogs need their "tribe" as much as people do.

- **Continuing with your workouts** will keep your endorphins pumping to stabilize your mood while expanding your pool of possible friends.

- **Entertainment** rituals give us time to de-stress. For years, before I left Austin, a dear friend and I went to a movie nearly every Sunday. The movie was only part of the process. Sundays can be particularly difficult if you're single, experiencing empty nest, loss of a mate or for other reasons. Alice and I saw some really awful movies, but they were still fodder for discussion, not to mention the popcorn and cokes that were part of the package. For you it could be a play, good blue-grass music, football, or hunting, but re-instating it is a source of comfort and satisfaction.

- **Morning coffee** at your own place certainly helps, but finding a neighborhood coffee shop where you'll meet new folks does double duty.

- **Weekly church/temple or meditating** helps keep us grounded and focused on our larger purpose. Very soon after moving in, create at least one room or space in the house where things feel calm and orderly and to which you can retreat for a moment of sanity in the prevailing chaos that characterizes moving.

- **Gardening,** for those who do it as part of their routine, is an out-let for creativity and a means of grounding. If you've brought a plant or two from your previous garden, take some special time to find just the right place for it in your new garden as a symbol of your "putting down roots." I have always had the need to *make the yard mine.* In the same way that home expresses and influences our personality, so does landscaping.

Simple Awareness

We often go through our days with such automation that we are hardly aware of all the things we do that give meaning to life. Whether moving to a new place or simply into a new phase, taking time to pay attention can be a renewing and grounding experience. Eastern traditions and philosophies put great store in the act of being *present* or *mindful,* which in-and-of itself is a meditation. In the act of focusing only on what is happening in the present moment, we become aware of sounds, colors, sensations and feelings in a way that eludes us when we are always multi-tasking and thinking about what we need to do next. Taking a deep breath, feeling our feet planted on the earth and noticing what we are doing give us insight into what has meaning and what is simply filling time.

The process of moving takes everyone off into ten different directions at once and we lose sight of priorities, relationships, and ourselves. Take a moment whenever you can and say hello to yourself, really make eye contact with the parent you are helping, and realize the gift of the moment. It is truly a gift to be part of the conscious process of designing the next stage of life and bringing it into realty.

Rituals and Ceremonies

Clearing the House

This is a ceremony I've been doing for years and it is both a cleansing and a blessing. My personal preference is to bless a space only after I have rid it of stale energy. As with any ritual, the real work is done with your intention. The motions, candles, incense and prayers or chants are really a way of holding *the space.* They help us focus our attention on the process and not get pulled off into irrelevant thoughts—the grocery list, wondering who lived here last or who will buy it. Ritual is also a way of separating us from the past history of the house or our fears about the future. This is really important, because the emotion you carry with you into the ritual defines the energy. You want to intend only the best and that which is for the highest and best good in the situation. This is a self-less process and is your connection to your higher self and whatever you consider divine energy.

I've used the following ritual for years. It is not affiliated with any particular religion but contains components of many different practices, some of which you may recognize.

What you will need:

- Sea Salt or Epsom salts;

- Wood alcohol (rubbing alcohol);

- One or more small containers such as a small saucepan or condiment dishes;

- Frankincense and Myrrh incense;

- A bell, drum, singing bowl—or hands for clapping.

What you will do:

- The Burn starts the process.

- Place about a half an inch of salt into your container;

- Pour just enough alcohol over the salt to create a film over the top;

- Place the mixture in the center of the house, or several scattered about the space;

- Make sure there are no flammable fumes in the house, fans are turned off and pets and children are out of the room. (Cats' tails are quite flammable you know...);

- Light the mixture and allow it to burn out (about 5 minutes usually does it).

Clearing with sound

- Sound your bell, bowl or drum, or clap your hands while walking around the house in a clockwise direction, moving in a clockwise direction in each room while getting to each of the corners. Let the quality and clarity of the sound guide you. Areas with stagnant energy will sound muted or muddy. Repeat those areas.

- While sounding, you may say your own version of a prayer or affirmation aimed at clearing all old energy and returning it in the enlightened state. My preference is a Buddhist chant that is part of the Heart Sutra and is goes like this:

"Gate gate, paragate, parasahmgate, bodhi swaha."

One approximate translation of this Sanskrit mantra is: "gone, gone" (gate, gate), "altogether gone" (or "gone without remnant") (paragate), "altogether gone to the other side" (or "gone without remnant and crossed to the other side"). I use it because I like the ritualistic nature of it, the sense of history and its long association with cleansing the heart of all emotions that are not useful and for one's highest and best good. It also keeps my mind focused on the process, not allowing it to drift into emotions that do not support my process.

- End at the spot where you started and express your gratitude for this clearing.

Blessing with Incense

- Light your incense.

- Starting at the front door, walk a path through the house again;, this time making sure the incense smoke gets into the corners, closets and recesses of the space.

- While walking, hold the intention that the house be filled with light, love, health and wellbeing. I repeat another Buddhist chant for this stage: *"Om mani pad me hum."*

The literal translation of this mantra is said to be "the jewel is in the lotus," which is filled with meaning in the practice of Buddhism, but difficult to explain in western terms. The essence of this mantra is the embodiment of wisdom, loving kindness and compassion for all beings.

- When you are complete, offer your gratitude and respectfully put away your blessing tools.

I use a more involved process than the one above, but this or a similar ritual of your own design will work. Remember, it is the reverence and intention with which the process is offered that is effective. Don't be surprised if you are overcome with emotion, sense the presence of angels, guides or the spirit of loved ones. This is a truly powerful practice that has been used for thousands of years in some variation and it connects you to a greater universe.

Further, you don't have to be present for the blessing to feel the difference in the space afterward. I performed a space clearing for a real estate company following a contentious partnership dissolution. The owner knew when the clearing would be done and she told no one. The morning after the clearing and blessing, agents commented on how different the place felt—wondering if something was cleaned, painted or moved. Moods changed and camaraderie returned. In another instance, a client reported that he slept better and that the home felt lighter and cleaner.

Simple Blessing

Another approach to clearing and blessing could be as simple as purchasing enough white candles to go in every room. Light the candles while playing some meditation music. Sit in the center of the house and visualize your beautiful life while living there. According to the research done in Quantum Physics and healing, visualizing it for you parent is just as powerful as their doing it for themselves. Our own loving intentions for another person are powerful beyond belief.

Exterior Blessing

There is an ancient and quite complicated rice blessing, requiring two minerals found typically only in Chinese apothecaries. Since uncooked rice is dangerous for birds and the minerals are poisonous, requiring that much care must be taken to wash the hands and keep them out of the reach of animals, I recommend an eco-friendly version using bird seed. Since intention is at the core of any blessing, bird seed works. Rice was used in Asian tradition because it represented the ability to feed and nourish your family. The more rice a family had, the more abundant it was considered.

What you will need:

A package of birdseed of your choosing. What doesn't get eaten will probably sprout.

What you will do:

- Recite: *Om madi pad me hum* while stirring ingredients in with middle finger pointed down (for grounding).

- Start at the front door.

- Scatter seed around the foundation or property boundary in the following sequence:
  - 3 handfuls—palm up expelling unwanted energy;
  - 3 handfuls palm down: planting the seeds of new growth, blessings and opportunity;
  - 3 additional handfuls up in the air with *Om mani pad me hum.*

- You don't have to do entire exterior if the property is in a complex.

Create Your Own

The most important elements of any blessing or ritual are your mindfulness in creating it, your ability to maintain focus while performing it and the good will you hold in your heart. I call this *holding the space*, and anything that is meaningful to you can fulfill that purpose.

An example comes to mind with my niece, then about seven years old and spending the night in a room she identified as "scary." (Admittedly there had been more than a few ghost reports in that room, though none had been shared with her.) Rising to the occasion to clear out the spooky feeling and get her comfortable with the space, we grabbed a few drums and bells, did a little dance around the room with her and just for good measure sprinkled lemon water around the room and in the corners. It was fun and she felt totally happy about the room and went fast asleep.

Months later, something unhappy occurred in her own home and when her mother mentioned it, Sarah suggested they dance around with noise makers and sprinkle lemon juice to make it feel better. And that is the way rituals are born...

Summary and Major Points

1. Each of us has rituals (habits) that play an important role in feeing grounded and comfortable in daily life.

2. When those habits or rituals are interrupted, we can feel adrift and without direction.

3. These rituals become more important when routine is disrupted, especially when other familiar aspects of life have been removed, as in the case when we move.

4. Recreating those rituals when relocating helps with re-establishing a sense of home and becoming emotionally connected.

5. Other rituals, which are consciously created, can be ways to show our commitment to a place, a concept, a relationship, or a process.

6. When leaving our established home, it can be a helpful part of the process to consciously say good-bye to the space, and honor the memories and life we experienced together (as we would with an old friend), before moving on.

7. When moving into the new home, cleansing and blessing the house energetically is as important as cleaning it physically. Doing this is the equivalent to cleaning a used artist canvas, before starting a new painting.

8. Housewarmings help us fill the new space with possibility and are a wonderful way to connect your parents with their new home and community.

9. As soon as possible, help your parents start re-establishing their daily rituals in the context of their new home.

Suggested Activities

1. Spend some time with your parents and explore what daily activities and rituals are important to them (morning coffee, a walk, reading the paper, prayer, walking their pet, etc.).

2. With your parents, begin to think about ways to re-incorporate those into their new routine as quickly as possible.

3. Make a list of items you might want to pack and take with you in the car, to be able to have them available immediately upon arrival at their new home.

4. If your parents' move is taking them far from their current home town, talk with them about the people or places they need to visit before leaving. This is a good opportunity to see if they would like to participate in a ritual (or a farewell party) in their home to honor the time spent there.

5. What rituals would you like to help your parent create, either for them or for you, if such a practice will help either of you to move forward?

13

Special Needs for Your Aging Parent

No discussion of moving later in life is complete without offering solutions to the variety of special needs that frequently arrive during this stage. The questions posed in this book are relevant for any move, especially those after the age of sixty, and will go far in addressing many special needs, but the following information is really designed for situations where health issues go beyond "normal aging." Very often, loved ones can remain in their homes or in independent living communities with minor adjustments made to their environments. Many of the frustrations, accidents and vulnerabilities we see among those in their 70s and beyond are directly related to issues that can be easily addressed if we can just identify the problem. The first hurdle is awareness of those needs, and if they have come on gradually—as they usually do —the person in need may not be able to identify the problem or articulate the specific adjustments that need to be made.

This chapter will offer adjustments that come from my own experience as an Audiologist working with clients with hearing loss, the experiences with my mother, the lessons learned from the many clients with whom I have worked, and recommendations from the American Academy of Occupational Therapists and the Alzheimer's Association.

Before we can determine adjustments, we obviously need to identify the specific needs. Frequently challenges occur well before a need is identified as a disability, or is obvious to the casual observer. Hearing loss is a classic example that is not always identifiable, except for our realization that "Dad isn't tuned in," or because he answers the wrong question or asks people to repeat. Vision is another. Before cataracts become serious enough to be visible to others, or operable, glare becomes an issue. Additionally, there are a few situations that are not true disabilities, just normal changes related to aging.

We'll begin by looking at symptoms and offer a few questions that might help you identify areas where adjustments can make life easier, safer and more carefree. Because we are most often alerted to special needs in the course of going about our daily routines, questions are related to schedules, routines and habitual functioning. The larger goal is to integrate adjustments into the normal environment to allow those who need them to live as normally and gracefully as possible.

Daily Routines

Dressing

- **Do they have the right container for their clothing?** Everyone needs a drawer for underwear, socks, a hanging place or drawer for trousers, skirts, dresses, coats. I know this seems obvious, but many of the problems associated with people feeling out-of-order relates to not having storage pieces that work. Check out the obvious first.
  - o **Solution:** Provide **adequate** drawer or hanging space. Unless there is a compelling reason otherwise (things need to be kept visible), I don't recommend shelving for foldable items because stacked items tend to shift and they are hard to maintain.
- **Can he/she identify where to put things?** Alzheimer's and dementia interfere with both memory and identifying the meaning of words, symbols, and uses.
  - o **Solution:** Label drawers with typed large print labels, pictures or knobs that identify the contents. Fun and beautiful knobs showing clothing items, tools, etc. are available from high-end hardware stores and catalogs. Transparent drawer fronts are another remedy.
- **Are clean and dirty clothes separated? If not, why not?**
  - o **Solution:** Perhaps all they need is a hamper that fits the space and is placed where they undress. Walking into another room to deposit clothes when you're already fatigued or aching with arthritis, or have mobility or vision problems, doesn't work.

- **Is there a place to hang up clothes easily, without having to create space?** If strength in hands and arms is reduced (arthritis, lack of exercise, atrophy), having to fight a stuffed closet results in clothing piling up on floors and furniture, making it difficult to find things, doing excess laundry, and general messiness that contributes to confusion and depression.

    o **Solution:** The simple solution is to either move seasonal clothes to another closet, purge outgrown clothes, those that are hard to get into (zippers they can't reach, buttons that are too small for arthritic hands, pull-over clothing they can't manage, etc). The installation of **double-decker** racks can improve access. Replacement of single garment hangers with those that accommodate multiple pairs of slacks, skirts, blouses or scarves help can increase maneuvering room.

- **Is the closet well lit?** Older eyes take in less light than they used to. Adequate light is essential to reduce frustration and help them match items.

    o **Solution:** Use higher wattage bulbs and arrange blacks and navy clothing nearer the light source to ease identification. Alternating dark items with lighter colored clothing can help, as well as pairing of sets by someone else.

- **Are the hanging racks placed at a level they can manage?** Range of motion needs to be considered.

    o **Solution:** Lower hanging racks and/or place some clothing in drawers.

- **Are drawers placed at the proper level** to avoid painful bending or reaching, and can they be opened and closed with ease?

    o **Solution:** Place the most used items at the easiest to reach position and store off-season items in others drawers. Dispense with habitual arrangements and create storage that works for the situation.

- **Do they have difficulty zipping, buttoning, pulling up socks, or slipping into shoes?**

○ **Solution:** Whenever possible, replace items with easier-to-manage clothing. Otherwise, many personal help items can help with routine dressing tasks. Items for pulling up socks, zipping, bracelet fasteners, etc. are available from catalogs listed in the back of this book.

- **Do they FEEL good in the clothing they have?** Colors, style and comfort are hugely important and are often forgotten when more physical problems may seem more pressing. Cheerful colors and styles lift the spirits and therefore can boost the immune system. Don't overlook style and color just because your parent never leaves her home or because he/she has "perfectly functional clothing." Attractive clothing can be found everywhere now: resale shops, discount stores and charities.

  ○ **Solution:** Go through their clothes with them and help them to let go of gloomy colors and styles. It's better to have fewer items than wear things that make us look and feel sick at heart. However, a word of warning! Clothing is so personal, it's easy to be intrusive. The goal here is for your parents to have clothing that is not only comfortable, and easy for them to button, etc., but clothing that they feel happy wearing.

Meals

- **Do they cook for themselves or want to?** If yes, do they have items on hand that are easy to open and prepare?

  ○ **Solution:** Shop for healthy mixes or partially prepared items that can easily be readied. Stick a list of these on the frig door to help your parent remember that they have these foods. This will promote better eating habits.

- **If so, how do they accomplish shopping, storage, etc.?** Do they need transportation help from a neighbor, family member, friend or service?

  ○ **Solutions:** CARTS, local taxis, volunteer transportation if available. As mentioned before, many grocery stores now deliver without charge.

- **If they do not cook, would a service like Meals on Wheels be appropriate, or can family members help?**
  - Solution: Family members or friends can prepare a few days' worth at a time and separate them into plates that can be warmed as needed. Nutritional snacks can be purchased in bulk and kept available and visible in baskets, near their bed or favorite chair.
- **Do they need help getting to and from the store or getting items from the car into the house?**
  - Solution: Carriers or rearranging the kitchen might help. Smaller grocery bags, with balanced loads or handles that can be more easily managed, help to maintain independence.
- **If they cook, can they easily lift heavy pots and pans and china?** Some items are just too heavy to lift with arthritic or weak hands and wrists.
  - Solution: Replace heavy items and those with small handles with more user-friendly varieties. Beautiful dishes can now be found in non-breakable, dishwasher-safe plastic. Double handles can be helpful.
- **Is the pantry organized and illuminated in such a way that they can easily reach and see items?**
  - Solution: Higher wattage bulbs, tap lights, turntables, bins and pull-out shelves can help with visibility. A professional organizer or closet planner can be enlisted if needed.
- **Do they need rails around the stove to prevent them from spilling (Parkinson's Disease for example)?**
  - Solution: An occupational therapist can help with strategies and planning. Rails or frames can be added to counter tops as they are on ships.
- **Can they easily access pots and pans?**
  - Solution: Plates may always have been shelved at eye level and pots and pans below counters, but this is no reason to keep it that way. Find alternatives that match flexibility, dexterity, and vision needs. Deep drawers for pots and pans can be retro-fitted

into an older kitchen as can many other user-friendly modifications.

- **Is the cook surface safe?** Are the knobs easy to read and turn on and off? Is there a tendency to leave pots on an electric surface, creating a fire hazard?
  - o **Solution:** Use of a microwave for heating, **or** the use of colored marks or stickers to identify settings. Larger knobs, easy-to-read stick-on labels made with colored label-maker tape increase safety.

- **Do they have access to nutritious snacks** (to maintain energy and blood sugar levels) that they can easily find and open to help maintain proper blood sugar and cognition? Both mood and mental processing are impacted by water and nutritional intake.
  - o **Solution:** Bottled water or easy access to quality drinking water and high quality, nutritional snacks. If opening a snack is problematic, unwrap a week's worth and store them in airtight containers or Zipper bags that they can open more easily. Be sure there are kitchen scissors available for stubborn packages, too.

Personal Hygiene

- **What is their level of self-care? If they are not taking care of self, identify the problem. Some possibilities are:**
  - Poor access;
  - Reduced vision (can't see the problem at hand);
  - Poor sense of smell;
  - Depression;
  - Lack of energy;
  - Lack of motivation;
  - Belief that no one cares;
  - Soap irritates their skin;
  - Modesty;
  - Fear of slipping in tub or shower;
  - Forgetting to bathe.
  - o **Solution:** determine the problem and find non-allergenic soap, provide a bath stool or railing, or a walk-in shower, provide a shower curtain or stall cover, provide for nursing help if necessary, and compliment them on how they look and let them know their appearance and health matters.

- **Is the bathroom floor slip resistant?**

- **Solution:** Textured tile is better than ceramic; non-slip backing on a heavy area rug is more stable than a flimsy bathmat; replaceable carpet is a quick alternative.

- **Can they safely navigate the bathroom and tell what's positioned where**? Some vision problems result in lack of depth perception, a problem that is exacerbated in most bathrooms because of the monochrome color pattern and high gloss surfaces.
  - **Solution:** Choose a colored toilet seat cover or contrasting colors for floor, tub, toilet, sink, etc. The greater the color contrast, the easier it is to find things.

- **Can they easily open and close cabinet doors?**
  - **Solution:** Choose large knobs, deep handles or levers to accommodate arthritis or swollen fingers.

- **Is there kick-space under cabinets** to allow for getting close to the sink or appliance?
  - **Solution:** Raise cabinets at least 3 inches off the floor or provide room for chair for sitting while applying make-up, shaving, and other hygiene tasks.

- **Are soaps and shampoos safely in reach?**
  - **Solution:** wall-mounted dispenser can be easier to handle, as can soap-on-a-rope.

- **Are towels/make-up/and other hygiene items easily accessible?**
  - **Solution:** Open cabinets, racks or hooks make the bathing ritual easier, and keep towels handy and off the floor.

- **In choosing a new space, is there maneuvering room for a walker or wheel chair if needed?**
  - **Solution:** Doorways should be at least 36" wide for wheel chair or **walker** access. Full circle turning diameter is 60".

- **Do they have difficulty getting up from a seated position?**
  - **Solution**: A raised **toilet** seat or wall-mounted handrail might be helpful. Padded seats can also be helpful for bony frames or fragile skin.

- **Can they find the bathroom at night without turning on a light?** Turning on a bright light can interfere with night vision and increase the possibility of a fall or disorientation.

       ○ **Solution:** Use a night-light, tap-light or low wattage lamp.

Sleeping

- **Is the bedroom arranged for maximum privacy and safety?**
  - ○ **Solution:** See Chapter 9, Diagram 1. Provide room for a walker or wheelchair when necessary. Provide a floor covering free of bumps and ridges. Preferences for foot movement vary: some prefer carpet for non-slip properties, other want a smooth surface because they *can* slide their feet.

- **Is incontinence or urgency an issue?**
  - ○ **Solution:** position the bed near the bathroom, but preferably not in *view* of the toilet or in line with the bathroom door. Seeing the toilet from the bed isn't particularly pleasing and it can actually increase the frequency of urination because of the subconscious reminder. However, Alzheimer's or dementia patients may need to *see* the toilet to remember where it is. A bedside commode could be a possibility.

- **Can they get in and out of bed easily?**
  - ○ **Solution:** The optimum height can be managed with extra deep or shallow mattresses, adjustable bed frames, or bed lifts available through catalogues and stores like the Container Store.

- **A reading lamp is a necessity, but its placement should be ergonomic.**
  - ○ **Solution:** Attach the lamp to the wall at a reachable height if knocking it   over (fire hazard) is a possibility. If dexterity is a problem, consider a lamp with a pull chain, toggle switch, or tap light.

- **Bedside access to essentials is a must.**
  - ○ **Solution:** Table should be sturdy and large enough to accommodate phone with auto dial for emergency numbers OR a list typed in large print, easy to read without glasses; also Kleenex, medications, reading material.

- **Is there a history of falling?**

- o **Solution:** Furniture should have round edges or corner protectors, which can be purchased from baby-proofing departments.

- **Is there a difficulty with comfortable sleep positions?**

  - o **Solution:** Install a foot cage if pressure on the feet is a problem, or simply leave the bedcovers un-tucked at the foot of the bed. **Pillows** for positioning can help reduce pressure on knees, back, neck, and hips. There are pressure-relieving mattresses that are now routinely used in nursing homes for vulnerable residents.

- **Is sleep interrupted by outside noise?**

  - o **Solution:** Consider either moving the bed/bedroom, or using a white noise generator to mask sleep-depriving sounds. Moving the bed away from walls that share the bathroom, utilities, air-conditioner, or kids' room may   be all it takes to promote a good night's sleep. If street noise and light are problematic, consider room darkening and sound insulating drapes, or moving to a different room.

Entertainment

- **Can they operate the TV and video/CD player?**

  - o **Solution:** Colored dots made with stick-on tape or fingernail polish can help identify buttons. Type out a large-print cheat-sheet for them.

- **Are others in the house (or neighbors) bothered by the volume on the TV or stereo?**

  - o **Solution:** Consider the pillow type amplifier or other personal assisted-listening device that only the user can hear.

- **Is there a glare on the TV screen or elsewhere in the room that interferes with lip-reading?** Even if a hearing loss is not obvious, many marginally impaired listeners need the redundancy afforded by lip reading, and glare is a real interference.

  - o **Solution:** Arrange the room to limit glare on the TV screen and elsewhere in the room. TV cable inlets can be relocated at little expense. Matte finishes on countertops can reduce glare. Adjustable window coverings, and sheer drapes can soften the light.

Harsh overhead lighting can be replaced or softened by task light-ing with soft white or full-spectrum or balanced spectrum bulbs.

- **Do they have easy access to the things that give their life mean-ing?**
  o A table for doing jigsaw puzzles;
  o A bookrack for holding crossword reference books;
  o Basket for keeping needlework handy;
  o Needlework frame with magnifying light for doing cross-stitch or needle point;
  o Large print books for reading;
  o Readers for books for the blind;
  o Books on tape and necessary equipment;
  o Pictures of grandkids near;
  o Letter writing materials;
  o Pets if desired;
  o An e-mail station for keeping in contact with kids and grandkids?

- **Do they have an EASY to operate e-mail station in case kids and grandkids want to e-mail**? Computers are alien to many older adults, and despite not being able to keep in touch, many folks, my mother included, just will not use a standard computer.
  o **Solution:** An easier to use e-mail only station might be the an-swer to keeping in touch. Those offering video viewing can be fa-bulous for keeping in touch with growing grandkids living far away.

- **Do they have access to gardening, if that's been an interest?**
  o **Solution:** If they can no longer get into the yard, planters can be positioned at chair height on decks that allow easy access. Some retirement communities have community gardens where resi-dents can grow flowers or vegetables to make this pastime possi-ble. In others, some planting is allowed around individual units.

- **Birdwatchers need to be able to watch their birds from a com-fortable spot and to be able to feed the birds.**
  o **Solution:** Window, deck and feeder access can be made possible through platform feeders, feeders on pulleys or window feeders.

Locate local groups and determine what level of activity is needed for outings.

Barrier-Free Considerations by Specific Impairment

Hearing Impairment

Hearing impairment is one of the more difficult disabilities to deal with because it is not visible. At first glance, one might wonder what this particular disability has to do with barrier-free design, inasmuch as it doesn't impair mobility and physical functioning in the ways we associate with other disabilities. Contrary to popular understanding, however, hearing-impaired clients can be helped enormously by modifications to their physical environment.

Some background regarding hearing loss might help. The type of hearing loss most often associated with aging and disability is known as a sensory-neural loss or nerve loss. It is characterized by:

- Inability to hear consonants, resulting in speech sounding garbled even if loud enough;

- Excessive sensitivity to noise.

> What is not often understood about hearing loss is why speaking louder won't always help and how someone who can't hear most sounds can be overly sensitive to sounds that don't bother someone with normal hearing.

The answer comes in two parts.

First, the type of loss characteristic of aging is called presbycousis, and it results from deterioration of nerves in the inner ear, which causes loss of acuity in the high frequencies. This is important, because the loss of acuity is accompanied by sound distortion that no amount of amplification can correct. Therefore, individuals with hearing loss may hear the vowel sounds (lower frequencies), which alert them to the fact that someone is speaking, but not be able to understand, because they are missing the consonant sounds that give it intelligibility. So the word "lunch" might be heard as "unh," or "Could you pass the spinach please? heard as "_oodu__ah__in__ eee." You can see why it's hard to carry on a conversation this way. Add background noise and you have a recipe for failure.

Second, the same nerve damage that causes poor comprehension can also make a high-pitched whistle excruciating and hearing aids impossible to wear in noisy situations.

Behavioral characteristics may include any/ all of the following:

- Misunderstanding what people are saying even if they are speak loudly enough;
- Inappropriate responses to questions and conversation;
- Failure to hear warning sounds;
- Can't talk on phone, understand TV;
- Isolating themselves from community;
- Pain and/or irritability with "normal" sounds;
- Extreme sensitivity to noise;
- Understanding of men's voices more easily than women and children.

Hearing aids are not always the answer and DO NOT change the fact that nerves are damaged. Speech will always sound like it's coming through a broken speaker. Therefore, visual cues are paramount. Reading lip movements and facial cues are a requirement for most hearing-impaired people and both comprehension and socialization improve with:

- Reduced glare;
- Good lighting;
- Reduced background noise;
- Sitting with the bright light or glare behind them;
- Sitting away from high traffic areas;
- Full face or profile view of the speaker(s).

Because of their inability to hear clearly and respond appropriately, many individuals with hearing loss dread family functions and group events where many people are talking at once, lots of background noise, and the inability to clearly see the person speaking to them. A family dinner becomes a nightmare, UNLESS: they are seated at the end of the table (away from the kitchen and high noise patterns, AND able to see people on both sides of table at least in profile. I can remember the dramatic difference in enjoyment when we sat Mom at the end of the table at a large Thanksgiving dinner. She was able to understand most of what was said to her and carry on a conversation that was consistent with her intelligence.

Environmental Adjustments for Hearing Impairment

PROBLEM	GOAL	SOLUTION or RATIONALE
Glare	• See low vision adjustments	• Improved lip reading
Speech Comprehension	• Carpet (low/hard pile) • Acoustic insulation around noisy appliances • Position conversational seating away from laundry • People should face the listener when speaking • Lower volume of background music & TV when communicating	• Reduce background noise
Safety	• Flashing, vibrating alarms for telephone, door bell, and fire	• Visual and tactile alerting

Low Vision

Low vision is a severe chronic visual impairment, which affects about 1 in 6 adults over 45 years of age and is the third leading cause of disability of aging, preceded by cardiac disease and arthritis. In an older population, it is caused primarily by glaucoma, diabetic retinopathy or macular degeneration.

Situational complications: vision can change depending on a number of situational characteristics:

- Lighting changes;

- Peripheral field limitations;

- Lack of color contrast;

- Background noise: mental drain, distracts the senses, fatigues;

- Depth perception issues;

- Movement.

Impact on daily life spans the most basic of activities required to maintain independence:

- Grooming;

- Judging depth of stairs and curbs;

- Monitoring medical requirements;

- Dialing emergency numbers;

- Identifying dials on stoves, household controls, spills;

- Judging distance/heights in bathroom and monochrome environments;

- Meal preparation;

- Avoidance of activities like reading, sewing, previously enjoyed hobbies, close-work.

Environmental Adjustments for Low Vision

PROBLEM	GOAL	SOLUTION or RATIONALE
General	• Task lighting at desk and in kitchen	• Improve visibility
	• Motion sensor lights at entrances	• Prevent falls
	• Lights at top and bottom of stairs	• Prevent falls
	• Contrasting colors in bathroom towel colors contrast with wall color	• Delineate tub and floor and help finding towels
	• Toilet seat cover for color contrast	• Find toilet
	• Under-counter lighting	• Improve visibility
	• Stair strip with contrasting color	• Prevent falls
	• Knobs/fixtures that contrast with doors	• Location & better grasp
	• Tap lights near bed or in darkened areas	• Safety
	• Experiment with the type of lighting that works best for client	• Safety, visual comfort
	• Accessible wall-mounted flashlights	• Safety and accessibility
	• Reduce background noises	• Improved sensory focus
	• Contrasting tape on outdoor steps and curbs	• Prevent falls
Glare	• Matte surfaces on counter tops	• Comfort/visibility/ safety
	• Glare reducing fabrics and wall coverings	• Comfort/visibility
	• Light fixtures/shades that control glare	• Comfort, lip-reading
	• Seating with light BEHIND client for enhanced lip reading	• Enhanced lip-reading
	• Window coverings that allow subtle control of outside lighting	• Safety, improved lip-reading
	• Carpet or runners on shiny floors	• Safety
	• Embedded glare-reduction treatments in window glass	• Improved visibility

Parkinson's Disease

Parkinson's Disease clients demonstrate a broad range of type and severity of symptoms, with tremor and muscle involvement interfering with everything from opening the mail to moving through the house. Environmental adjustments include, but are not limited to, the following:

Environmental Adjustments for Parkinson's Disease

LOCATION	GOAL	SOLUTION or RATIONALE
Bedrooms	• Clutter free • Stable furniture • Simple bed access/egress • Easy movement within bed • Easy access to bathroom • Chair with armrests • Raised seats • Satin sheets • Nightlights marking paths • Bell or intercom by bed	• Easy access storage • Remove casters / wheels • Bed rails/trapeze/bed pull • Bed cradle to lift covers off • Bed placement • Aids with dressing • Aids in rising from seat • Reduces friction in turning • Accident avoidance • Safety
Bath	• Non-skid tubs/floor • Large rugs instead of bath mat • Tub/shower seats • Shower wands • Grab bars • Curtain instead of glass doors • Hot water at 120 degrees max • Raised toilet seat • Soap-on-a-rope	• Prevents falls • Reduces tripping • Safer and easier bathing • Safer and easier bathing • Safety/ease of access • Safety/ease of access • Prevent scalding • Easier sitting/rising • Convenience/safety
Kitchen	• Cutting boards with raised edges and suction cups • Built in revolving storage • Stove top pot stabilizers	• Safer food preparation • Ease of access • Safety/self maintenance

LOCATION	GOAL	SOLUTION or RATIONALE
Kitchen	• Countertop microwave	• Instead of stove; reduces danger of burns
	• Pull-out pan storage	• Reduces lifting
	• Table top guard rails	• Meal time safety
	• Appliance garages	• Reduced clutter
	• Glasses with "beer mug" handles	• Easier grip
Pathways	• Avoid placing furniture at edge of corners/doors	• Reduce bruising
	• No furniture in hallways	• Avoids unsteady-gait injuries
	• Hallway handrails	• Improved ability to reach target
Fixtures	• Large, L-shaped levers	• Easier to grasp

Alzheimer's and Other Forms of Dementia

Alzheimer's is the leading form of dementia in America. Affecting not just memory, but personality and judgment as well, it presents environmental challenges not unlike those faced by Parkinson's patients and those with reduced vision, urinary incontinence and sleep disturbances. In general, the goal is to keep the environment as clear of obstruction as possible and reduce opportunities for injury related to falls, lack of coordination and poor judgment. A further problem is associated with the fact that one of the functions impacted by the disease is internal mapping, resulting in individuals becoming lost in their own home and neighborhood. Therefore, part of the goal with environments is to make it easier for them to identify their personal spaces and frequently used routes.

Since Alzheimer's is so prevalent and its progression can be delayed if treatment begins in the early stages, it's important to know the ten warning signs published by the Alzheimer's Association. More detailed information can be found at your local Alzheimer's Association and there are many excellent books on the topic. Among those that describe life with Alzheimer's patients, two excellent ones are *Elder Rage* by Jacqueline Marcell and *Talking to Alzheimer's* by Claudia J. Strauss.

Although some of these symptoms fall in the category of "normal aging," it's time to be concerned when difficulties continue to increase in frequency and severity and begin interfering with work, social activities and daily functioning. If you notice any of the Ten Warning Signs listed below in yourself or a loved one, it can be helpful to keep a notebook and take it with you if/when you consult a dementia specialist. To date, the drugs used to treat Alzheimer's can stall the progression, but cannot reverse the process.

The Ten Warning Signs of Alzheimer's

1. Memory loss;
2. Difficulty performing familiar tasks;
3. Problems with language;
4. Disorientation to time and place;
5. Poor or decreased judgment;
6. Problems with abstract thinking;
7. Misplacing things;
8. Changes in mood or behavior;
9. Changes in personality;
10. Loss of initiative.

Environmental Adjustments For Alzheimer's & Other Forms Of Dementia

LOCATION	GOAL	SOLUTION or RATIONALE
General	• Remove unnecessary furniture, rugs or obstacles	• Safety in walking
	• Replace glass tabletops with non-breakable	• Safety
	• Lighting easy to turn off/on	• Ease of operation
	• Enhanced lighting as in low vision	• Ease in finding things
	• Keep things simple and familiar	• Memory issues
	• Avoid strong patterns or contrasting block designs in flooring	• Causes disorientation and confusion
	• Paint critical entrances a different color	• Help with locating and remembering placements
	• Place objects that cue memory in plain view	• Helps them locate items and places
	• Store medications in lock box	• Prevent overdose

LOCATION	GOAL	SOLUTION or RATIONALE
General	• Consistent background noise/ music or nature sounds of their choosing • Create LARGE PRINT books with frequently asked questions and attach to favorite chair, bed side, bathroom • Identification bracelet with name, address, emergency phone contact	• Helps maintain calmness • Reduces answering same questions over and over, promotes calmness and independence • Locate family in case of wandering
Bedroom	• Rounded corners on bedside tables • Stow electric heaters, heating pads, and electric blankets • Arrange clothing in sequence and by season • Use pictures or labels for storage	• Prevent injury • Prevent burns / overheating • Helps with dressing appropriately • Locate/ stow belongings
Bath	• Remove curling irons, hair dryers • Clear countertops of clutter • Grab rails in tub, shower, near toilet • Shower or tub seat	• Safety • Safety; reduces confusion • Safety, ease with self care • Safety and hygiene
Kitchen	• Secure drawers with child-safety devices • Remove knobs from stoves/ heaters if access to those areas allowed • Provide sufficient lighting as in low vision and balance problems • High color contrast for eating utensils, drinking glasses and plates • Stow poisons, cleaning supplies	• Safety • Safety • Safety • Easy identification and access • Prevent poisoning

Summary and Major Points

1. Very often, loved ones can remain in their homes or in independent living communities if minor adjustments are made to their environments.

2. One way to become aware of the need for such adjustments is to become aware of symptoms that appear during the business of their going about daily life and the actions associated with the following activities:

- Dressing
- Meals
- Personal Hygiene
- Sleeping
- Entertainment

3. Specific questions are listed under each of the above categories to stimulate observation and awareness of the need to make adjustments to the environment.

4. Awareness of the symptoms associated with individual impairments can be stimulated by watching for the following behaviors or tendencies:

Hearing Impairment

- Misunderstanding what people are saying even if they are speak loudly enough;
- Inappropriate responses to questions and conversation;
- Failure to hear warning sounds;
- Can't talk on phone, understand TV;
- Isolating themselves from community;
- Pain and/or irritability with "normal" sounds;
- Extreme sensitivity to noise;
- Understanding of men's voices more easily than women and children.

Low Vision

- Poor grooming;
- Problems judging depth of stairs and curbs;

- Difficulty monitoring medical requirements;

- Difficulty dialing phone numbers;

- Trouble identifying dials on stoves, household controls, spills:

- Judging distance/heights in bathroom and monochrome environments:

- Messy or difficult meal preparation;

- Avoidance of activities like reading, sewing, previously enjoyed hobbies, close-work.

Parkinson's Disease

- Broad range of type and severity;

- Includes tremor and muscle involvement interfering with daily tasks from small motor activities like writing and opening the mail to walking, unsteady gait and generally poor muscle control.

Alzheimer's and other forms of Dementia:

- Memory loss.

- Difficulty performing familiar tasks.

- Problems with language.

- Disorientation to time and place.

- Poor or decreased judgment.

- Problems with abstract thinking.

- Misplacing things.

- Changes in mood or behavior.

- Changes in personality.

- Loss of initiative.

5. Environmental adjustments aimed at addressing specific problems and goals are provided for each of the limitations mentioned in the chapter.

Suggested Activities

1. Spend some time accessing the behavioral characteristics and list areas of difficulty with daily life exhibited by your parent(s):

2. Have a conversation with your parents to discuss their view of activities they find challenging and their ideas on what might help and list your findings below.

3. Review the Environmental Adjustment charts and make a list of those changes you can make in their existing home or the new residence.

4. What items, if any, will you need to purchase or get assistance with implementing?

14

Taking Care of Yourself

Our bodily systems can be challenged at many levels when we are involved in a major life event such as divorce, marriage, death of a loved one or helping another through any of these challenges. The effects on us can be mental, physical, emotional and spiritual. It takes special handling, not just for those for whom you are caring, but for yourself as well. In fact, before we can adequately take care of others, especially over the long haul, we *must* find ways to take care of ourselves. We've already talked about some of the conflicting emotions that arise during such an event. Those emotions can cause significant hormonal changes that impact our immune system and our ability to cope. So how do we go about taking care of ourselves, when so much chaos surrounds us?

There are the standards mentioned in every workshop and book: a long hot bath, dinner with a friend, a massage or manicure. All of these can help in the short term, but do little for the long-term day-to-day management of the deeper cause and results of stress. When you can manage to build in any of these small acts of kindness to yourself, I wholly recommend it. Some of these however require more time or financial resources that we have or want to contribute to this worthy cause. At times, getting a little "private time" seems to create more angst than it cures and we feel worse rather than better as the result of awarding ourselves such "guilty pleasures," even though they are precisely what we need to give us a little respite and distance.

While the above moments of self-care can help to take the edge off, there are others that have a deep and lasting impact. Among the possibilities are physical exercise, targeted movements to re-wire the brain, cleansing and recharging the body's energy engines, deep relaxation, frequent time-outs and FUN.

Among the tools I use and have taught others are several that are relied upon routinely by energy workers and healers. I've learned and applied these over the course of thirty years spent studying and working with the human energy field, and as a requirement for my being able to do the work I do. When I started doing healing work, Feng Shui and coaching years ago, it wasn't unusual for me to come home feeling totally depleted from expending all of my own energy stores and resources. I was literally giving my energy away, and recharging took time. I eventually learned to use my body as a conduit for the energy available to me and constantly recharge through a process of breathing and intention. For those who have never worked with this concept, it may sound foreign at first. It might help to think about tapping into an external source of energy by using the analogy of Scuba divers and their air tanks. If divers had to rely only on the air they could hold in their lungs to carry them through a dive over about three minutes, they would be out of air and out of luck fast. Instead, they carry with them a ready source of air (energy) to last them through a lengthy dive. We have just such a source of ready energy available to us—but even better than air tanks, this source is constantly renewable, coming as it does from the ambient field around us and through the process of conscious breathing, visualization and intention. These techniques will be addressed a little later.

I first came across this while taking a healing workshop with Barbara Brennan, Ph.D., author of *Hands of Lights* (1987) and other wonderful books on managing your own energy resources while using them to heal others as well as yourself. Since that time twenty years ago, it has been a staple in every other healer's training I've both taken and taught. It is the core of practices like Reiki, Pranic Healing, and Quantum Touch, all of which tap into and develop the practitioner's ability to use their own body as a conduit for energy they "transmit" to another. When I began using this technique in my work, I realized that I was actually energized at the end of the day. An added benefit was my ability to send energy to my client simultaneously. Clearing any negativity from my own mindset, setting healthy boundaries and charging have all become aspects of my own ritual before working with someone else, be it client or friend, and has become essentially automatic. On occasion, if I'm pre-occupied and bypass these practices, I notice a difference immediately and step back mentally and take care of myself before proceeding.

For those of you new to or only vaguely familiar with the concept of energy fields, ambient energy and hands-on healing, here's a short primer. (Those of you who feel you know this stuff, feel free to fast-forward.) We'll continue with the concepts introduced in Chapter Three where we talked about Quantum Physics and the principle of all matter as a mass of sub-atomic particles vibrating at different frequencies—and that includes our physical bodies. Just as our bodies are a mass of vibration, so does a field of higher vibrational energy surround us all. Most people cannot see this energy, called the *aura*, but those who can see and/or feel it describe this field as extending around us in roughly the shape of an egg or balloon. If we extend our arms straight out to each side, this bubble would extend a few inches beyond our fingertips, above the head and under our feet. (See Diagram 11).

The density, uniformity and integrity of this field of energy can impact and be impacted by forces within and beyond the body. It is generally accepted that disease starts first in the energetic field, before the symptoms show up in the physical body. By learning how to "feed and care for" this field, we can keep ourselves healthier, more grounded, calmer and more focused than is possible when operating by default. You've heard the word "scattered" used in reference to how we feel when we're doing too much and have portions of our attention and emotions fragmented while dealing with problems and events of the day. It's called *scattered and fragmented* precisely because we leave little "packets" of our energetic field with those people with whom we share an emotional bond—whether that's love, anger, worry, jealousy or sorrow. When we argue, love, worry and so on, there is a literal exchange of energy. In doing this, we have less emotional, intellectual and spiritual focus to bring to our own tasks. It's not that we draw from a limited field—that's infinite—but we have to learn to manage this field consciously to make best use of it. Techniques for doing this will appear later in this chapter, but for those of you who want to pursue this in greater depth, there are many excellent resources in the bibliography, including those by Barbara Brennan and Carolyn Myss

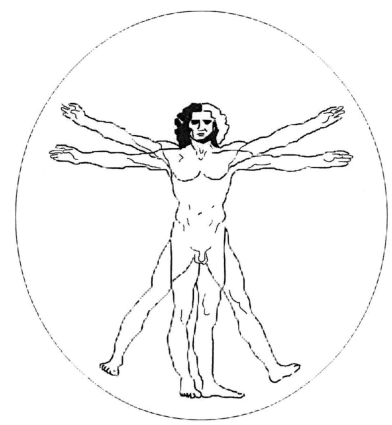

Diagram 11: The Aura and the Physical Body

What follows are some self-care tools that help with the event at hand. If used consciously in your normal routine, they will contribute enormously to your success in any endeavor you choose.

Water

Water is listed first because of its importance in overall health and well-being. You can do everything else right—eat, exercise, meditate, sleep—but if you don't drink enough water, the brain, the sole organ responsible for thinking, planning and negotiating all of these activities will not work properly. The human brain is approximately 75% water. Since the brain is essentially an electrical mechanism where neural impulses fire across synapses, conductivity is a central issue. Proper hydration is crucial to cognition and studies show that dehydration adversely affects thinking. A study cited in the International Journal of Psychophysiology revealed that under-hydration was related to slower psychomotor processing speed and reduced attention and memory among otherwise healthy older adults. Similar results were noted in a 2005 study conducted by the Pediatrics Unit at Soroka University Medical Center, Faculty of Health Sciences, Ben-Gurion University of the Negev, Ber Sheva, Israel.

Water consumption requirements vary depending on age, activity level, the heat index and a number of other factors addressed in exquisite detail in a 2004 International Life Sciences Institute (ILSI) Monograph. However, conventional wisdom is eight, eight-ounce servings per day—throughout the day, whether you're consciously thirsty or not. Don't substitute teas, coffee, sodas or alcohol for water, since they are diuretic and have an adverse effect. And remember that colds, allergies, or medications can cause dehydration, so drink extra water if any of those conditions exist.

Water is good for your brain, cellular health, kidney function, muscle integrity and mood. Lack of water not only negatively affects these functions, but can also contribute to back pain—and goodness knows, if you're packing and lifting boxes, you don't need any more of that...

Exercise and Movement

We know that exercise will help us lose those extra few pounds, bolster our immune system, improve cardiovascular health and keep us flexible and strong. Major life transitions are a Petri dish for stress, anxiety and depression, which can evolve into general malaise, disruption of sleep, digestive disorders and a multitude of other serious health concerns. What's important about exercise in terms of our topic has to do with the less talked-about benefits:

- Self-esteem;
- Improved energy;
- Endorphin output (mood enhancement);
- Physical and emotional strength;
- Improved sleep;
- Improved focus and problem solving ability;
- Greater sense of control over your life.

In the book, *The Power of Full Engagement* (Loehr and Schwartz, *2003)*, the subtitle says it all: "Managing Energy, Not Time, Is the Key to High Performance and Personal Renewal." We're talking about energy at all levels, not just physical energy, but it is important to note that a physical work-out regimen is an essential part of their program for corporate executives and others aiming for peak performance in all aspects of life. I offer a focused coaching program called *Integrative Living*. Its full value comes from integrating every life goal with every other and being fully engaged with each. Exercise is one aspect of life, which, if left out, shows up in all the others. The fact that you're lifting boxes and running yourself silly while moving Mom and Dad is not a substitute for regular resistance-training and aerobic exercise.

"What's good for the goose is good for the gander," or in this case, what's good for you can also be beneficial for your parent, even if suffering from a disease such as Alzheimer's. An article appearing in *Revolution Health*, originating from the Mayo Clinic, cited research showing that moderate exercise improves feelings of physical and emotional well-being for many people with Alzheimer's. Results indicated that as little as 20 minutes of walking three times a week can improve mood, decrease the number of falls, reduce wandering and even delay nursing home placement for people with Alzheimer's.

A generally agreed-upon approach to fitness includes daily exercise of a continuous nature for twenty to thirty minutes at a stretch, coupled with strength training to improve muscle mass, which improves oxygen and glucose utilization. This should be adjusted for age and physical ability. When we were younger, this level of exercise might have come from the type of work we did for a living, or from the activities we did for fun (sports, dancing, sex, hiking, bike-riding, skiing, etc.) Many of us lose touch with these activities through the process of building a career and family, injuries and loss of interest. The key later in life is to find something that is either fun, socially gratifying or an aspect of some other fulfilling activity, so that exercise is again integrated into the mainstream of our lives: dancing, gardening, hiking, yoga, tai chi, bicycling, Habitat for Humanity work, volunteer maintenance of a natural wilderness area and so on.

In addition to exercise, there are simple movements that can synchronize the left and right hemispheres and support mental activities so necessary in making the kinds of decisions necessary during this process. As mentioned in Chapter Five, different sides of the brain control different functions. The left-brain is strongly associated with more linear thinking, lists, and logical processes, while the right-brain is more global, creative and intuitive. Typically, we operate primarily from one side or the other, but seldom are they synchronized and functioning simultaneously. When they are, we have both the logical mind and the intuitive mind operating together, expanding our problem-solving ability and bringing two divergent functions together. Furthermore, the same physical movements that support brain synchronization stimulate areas of the brain that have to do with focus, categorizing, problem solving, emotion and impulse control.

All of these movements involve crossing the mid-line of the body. For example, when walking, the right arm naturally swings forward as the left leg steps forward. By moving the hand across the mid-line of the body when it swings, we are performing a cross-lateral movement.

Many activities such as knitting, dancing, swimming, walking, most sports (tennis, swimming, soccer, badminton), and playing a musical instrument such as the piano, violin or the drums involve movement of a hand or leg crossing the center line of the body. Therefore, they influence brain function in a specific manner that supports learning, memory and critical thinking.

Two excellent books that offer numerous very specific movements that stimulate the brain in even more targeted ways that support attention, memory, stress reduction, and thinking are: *Brain Gym* by Gail and Paul Dennison and *Smart Moves: Why learning Is Not All In Your Head* by Carla Hannaford.

Nutrition

Notice I didn't say diet here, because this is not about the kind of loathsome activity we participate in to lose weight. This is about feeling good, supporting the brain, having the energy we want to live the way we want, and feeling good in our bodies, whatever weight or body type we may exhibit. The contrary fact is that, for most of us, stress triggers a way of eating that absolutely sabotages us. The need for quick energy, emotional stroking, and the exposure to old patterns can drive even the most aware individual to binge on Little Debbie's and chips. Alcohol and other attempts at self-medicating add to our malaise. So, make it easier on yourself. Keep healthy snacks within reach; go *out* to have a piece of pie or cake and make it an occasion instead of having the whole dessert within arm's reach; find a few treats that mix healthy with a high "yummy" quotient (dark chocolate and nuts come to mind) and treat yourself well. Use the same list of foods recommended in Chapter 10 for support and snacks on moving day to provide the kind of overall eating pattern that will support body and brain throughout the move. If you're having trouble eating the recommended 7-13 servings of fruits and vegetables a day (and most of us are), I recommend Juice Plus, which "provides the nutrients of 17 different fruits, vegetables and grains in capsule form." It's not intended as a replacement for healthy eating, but it does support the published research shows that it supports the immune system.

The added benefit from these foods is that they both help you stay physically healthy, and contribute to optimum brain health as well. And the tool we use the most in the difficult decisions and emotions associated with life transition is the brain. If the brain isn't performing properly, all the physical strength in the world only gets us so far.

Deep Relaxation Practice or Meditation

The practice of deep relaxation, or the meditation process of your choice, has benefits beyond simply getting you to a more relaxed state of mind. Herbert Benson M.D. details his research on the biological impact of deep relaxation in his book, *The Relaxation Response,* and lists the following as just a few of the benefits:

- Decrease in the rate of oxygen consumption 10 - 20% within 3 minutes of reaching the relaxed state;

- Decrease in blood lactate (associated with anxiety) within 10 minutes of meditation;

- Decrease in the activity of the sympathetic nervous system associated with the fight or flight reaction;

- Lowering of blood pressure;

- Possible reduction in drug use;

- Reduction of blood sugars associated with insulin production and diabetes.

If you came of age during the time when Transcendental Meditation was the rage, you may have the idea that there's one way to meditate and if you're not doing it "right" it's not worth doing. So let's erase that idea. I appreciate the Buddhist phrase *sitting practice*, because it doesn't carry with it the rule set of having to clear your mind, have a personalized mantra and a myriad of other preconceived ideas or fears associated with the term "meditation."

Dr. Benson outlines a straightforward process, which will take you to a similar mental, emotional, spiritual place, but regardless of the method used, the basic components are the same. You'll need a relatively quiet place where you can get comfortable, an open and nonjudgmental attitude and an affirmation or thought, sound, or visual cue (like a candle) to return to when your mind wanders.

The Basic Technique:

- Sit quietly and uncross legs, ankles, arms and fingers;

- Close your eyes;

- Breathe deeply, slow belly-breaths (to the count of four in, four out for starters);

- Relax all muscles, starting with your feet and moving upward to your facial muscles, maintaining the relaxation;

- Continue breathing through your nose and be aware of your breathing;

- Continue sitting in this way for 15 - 20 minutes. Use your mental device to help keep focused if your mind wanders or fixates on a thought;

- Keep an open attitude. DON'T JUDGE yourself. Allow feelings, sensations, and thoughts to emerge. Be an observer.

If your mind wanders, and it probably will, because that's what minds do, try using a method known as "mindfulness meditation." It really is the best tool I've come across to conquer or at least quiet the "monkey brain," which goes off in all directions at once in response to a thought or distraction. It works like this. Say you're sitting quietly and out of the blue come the sounds of a distant motorcycle. The monkey-mind may wonder whose motorcycle it is, remind you of someone else's motorcycle and the last time you saw so-and-so, and where you went. That could take you to another related event and, well—that's the end of sitting quietly. Mindfulness meditation would have you simply identify the distraction as *sound* and have you return to your breathing or affirmation. You identify the distraction as something like sound, feeling, sensation, thought, etc., and therefore avoid the chase of the monkey-mind. It's a very effective tool and even the most practiced, experienced meditator confesses to a wandering mind. You might even suggest to yourself that these sounds, etc. will make you even more relaxed.

Some of the other benefits translate to being able to approximate this state of relaxation while fully alert, by use of a straightforward tactile association trigger. If, while meditating, you use a tactile trigger, like putting the thumb, index finger and middle finger together, it's possible to form a mental association between this state of relaxation and the trigger. Any time you want to access this deeper state of relaxation, even when you're in the midst of other activities, simply take a deep breath, put your fingers together and feel calmer, more centered and focused. Try this technique when you meditate and see how it works for you.

Strengthen Your Energy Field

Any time you want to feel stronger, more centered and energized, you can follow the method below.

- Close your eyes, take a few deep breaths and imagine you are in a bubble of white light. You can think of it like an egg or a balloon if it helps to see it in your mind.

- As you breathe in, imagine that you are taking in energy, breaths or light through all your pores. You can also imagine yourself in a column of white light starting from the heavens and surrounding you.

- As you exhale, visualize your egg or energy bubble getting larger and more dense as it expands. Get it to reach a two to three foot periphery around your body.

- Imagine that this bubble has a semi-permeable coating on it that is protective, and only positive energy can get through this "shell."

- Finally, whenever you feel yourself fatiguing, losing focus during your day or during your communications with someone, put your bubble in place and breathe into it.

- Practice this any time during the day, especially when you don't "need" it, so that it will feel natural to do this when you need to replenish your resources.

Note: Using this technique to establish your boundary can negate the need to establish it verbally. People sense your strength and integrity energetically and respond accordingly.

Reclaiming Your Energy

Use this technique whenever you've had an argument, done healing work, helped anyone with a task or emotion where you find that your thoughts are still with them, or feel they are draining your energy.

- Breathe into your energy bubble.

- Imagine an energy magnet running through the core of your body. (Remember when you were a little kid and worked with a horseshoe magnet and iron filings?)

- When this magnet is in place, recall your energy, and visualize it being drawn back to you by the powerful pull of this magnet.

- Intend that this energy be returned clean and ready for your use. You can visualize your aura filtering out anything it's collected along the way and returning only what belongs to you fresh and re-energized.

- Go about you day, knowing you have all of your resources at your disposal.

Establishing Boundaries

This is a useful technique whenever you feel the need to set healthier limits for yourself: when you need to "say no," protect yourself from hurtful sentiments expressed by others, or when others are needing more from you than you're prepared to give.

- Visualize your energy balloon, and strengthen its exterior shell.

- See yourself as being fully capable of establishing and maintaining your boundaries, and immerse yourself in the sensation of actually doing that. Set the intention that you will perform only those activities that *serve your ultimate goal.* It's possible that you have conflicting goals, and that's where many people have difficulty in setting the boundary. For example, you may want to reduce the number of requirements on your time and space (first intention), but you also want to keep harmony with your mother (underlying intention). It's important to understand at a deep level what your primary intention is. Then your choice or decision becomes more conscious and you're in control, rather than being controlled by an underlying agenda that hasn't come to awareness.

Chakras: Your Body's Power Centers

The body's energy centers through which life force flows are called Chakras. Literally translated as Wheels of Light, they were first identified in India as vortices of moving energy spinning at different rates. The function of the Chakras is to vitalize the body. Each is said to be "associated with an endocrine gland and major nerve plexus," (Brennan, *Hands of Light*, 1987). These centers of energy have recently been measured by Western medicine and shown to have a different level of electrical charge from other points in the body.

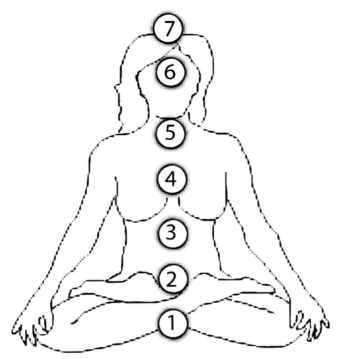

Diagram 12: Locations of the 7 Major Chakras

There are seven major Chakras along the centerline of the physical body (Diagram 12, and numerous minor Chakras elsewhere, including, but not limited to the palms of the hands and the soles of the feet. There are others external to the physical body, but for our purposes we'll work with the major seven Chakras and the first one external to the body. Each of first seven is associated with a color, within the range humans can discern. Each chakra relates to certain mental, physical and spiritual aspects, and can be thought of as a ladder starting at the base of the spine, and moving up through the body to just above the crown of the head. The base chakra, known at the Root, starts in the physical realm, with each successive rung taking us through the workings of the heart, then higher mind and the spirit, on to connection with divine consciousness.

When we feel bereft, fatigued, sluggish, scattered, unfocused, etc., it means energy is not moving through the body in a fluid manner and is "stuck" somewhere along the chain. If you've ever had Reiki or acupuncture or even a good massage, you may have experienced the sensation of movement from feet up through the body all the way to the scalp. You feel both energized and relaxed, grounded and in contact with spirit.

Think of your chakras as an energy battery. The chakras record and store information about life experiences, values and beliefs, with each one related to a specific category of information. Our physical and emotional health is related to whether we empower these energy centers or lose energy through negative associations.

1st Chakra is where we store information and rules about biological family, social history and culture. Our beliefs relate to our sense of survival, issues of loyalty, and identity.

- We *strengthen* the chakra when we live in integrity with beliefs that support us, nurture our connection with our environment, and maintain a connection with "family" or community.

- We can *weaken* the chakra by allowing others to dictate our rule base, when we act out of superiority or jealousy, and/or hold on to negative history and experiences with family.

2nd Chakra relates heavily to one-on-one relationships, and governs feelings about control, sex, money and personal power. Healthy and positive relationships require a connection between the second and fourth (heart) chakras.

- *Strengthening* this chakra can be accomplished through the release of past sexual traumas, nurturing relationships, and identification and release of addictive behaviors.

- The chakra is *weakened* when we attempt to control others, give into our fears about money, and hold onto unresolved conflicts about sexuality.

3rd Chakra has to do with maintaining boundaries we have chosen for ourselves (as opposed to those of the first chakra, which are mandated by our "tribe"), and our sense of personal power and esteem.

- We *empower* this chakra when we honor our "gut feelings," take pride in what we do and honor our commitments.

- *Loss of energy* occurs when we are inauthentic, ignore our intuitive voice, and allow others to violate our boundaries.

4th Chakra relates to the emotions and is the link that connects the upper three and lower three chakras. There is the indication that one cannot progress in spiritual development without involving the heart chakra, which houses information about love, forgiveness and harmony.

- *Empowerment* of this chakra involves allowing others to experience the world in their own way, forgiving with no strings attached, and self-love.

- *Depletion* occurs when we live with resentments or past grievances, degrade ourselves and fear success or moving forward.

5th Chakra has to do with finding our own voice. The second chakra had to do with power to control others; this one has to do with claiming our own power, getting ourselves "un-stuck," and making choices.

- *Support* comes through speaking authentically and honestly, exercising self-control, and using our voice to empower others.

- *Weakness* occurs when we fail to define our own needs and succumb to the will of others, speak dishonestly and experience shame.

6th Chakra is the seat of intellect and rational thought. Our spiritual evolution frequently demands that we open our minds to possibilities other than the rational.

- We can *energize* this chakra through honoring our intuition, taking emotional risks (non-rational) and dwelling in possibilities.

- *Blockages* occur when we fixate on the rational as a way to explain what we feel, hold on to old grief and become close-minded.

7th Chakra represents our connection with the divine in others and ourselves. It is the center for mysticism and a sense of grace. It relates to the skills of telepathy, seeing auras, out-of-body travel, healing and lucid dreaming.

- We can *heighten our energy* here through living with intention, meditation or prayer, living with gratitude and embracing each life experience as an opportunity to grow spiritually.

- *Loss of energy* occurs when we are disconnected from faith, refuse to listen to our higher self or guidance, unless the voice we hear comes from an "approved source."

8ᵗʰ Chakra, located about one foot above the top of the head, represents the energy of divine love, spiritual compassion and spiritual selflessness, karmic residue. It activates spiritual skills contained in the 7ᵗʰ chakra.

9ᵗʰ Chakra is the soul blueprint, the individual's total skills and abilities in all the lifetimes.

10ᵗʰ Chakra is our connection with divine creativity, synchronicity of life; merging of masculine and feminine within—unlocking the skills contained in the 9ᵗʰ chakra.

11ᵗʰ Chakra is the pathway to the Soul, the individual's ability to acquire advanced spiritual skills (travel to other dimensions, teleportation, bilocation, instantaneous perception of thoughts, telekinesis in some cases).

12ᵗʰ Chakra is our connection with source, understanding of and communication with the universe, the unlocking of the abilities of the 11ᵗʰ chakra.

The following chart offers some other common associations for Chakras 1 through 7.

Chakra	Color	Endocrine Gland	Psychological Function
7—Crown	Violet-White	Pineal	Spiritual connection
6—Brow	Indigo	Pituitary	Thought/intuition
5—Throat	Blue	Thyroid	Expression of will
4—Heart	Green	Thymus	Emotions
3—Solar Plexus	Yellow	Pancreas	Self Esteem
2—Sacral	Orange	Gonads	Personal power
1—Base	Red	Adrenals	Survival & Safety

Basic Chakra Cleansing

First find a quiet place and take a few deep, cleansing breaths like those in the Deep Relaxation Technique, and begin breathing into your energy balloon, or aura. This process will put you in the right frame of mind to focus and visualize the recharging of the basic seven chakras of the physical body.

Next, continue your breathing and visualization to include a column of light forming in the center of your body, from feet, along the general pathway of the spine, up through the neck and out of the top of your head and beyond to a level of about two feet above your head. The intention is to connect your practical, physical self to the divine, whatever that means for you personally.

The next few steps are repeated with each of the seven power centers:

1. Visualize the chakra as a ball of color about the diameter of a dinner plate:

- First—True red;
- Second—Orange;
- Third—Yellow;
- Fourth—Green;

- Fifth—Sky blue;
- Sixth—Indigo;
- Seventh—Violet-White.

2. If, when you visualize the color, it seems muddy or dark, continue holding the desired clear color in your mind. It's helpful to visualize a perfect Naval Orange for the color of the second chakra, a clear blue sky for the throat, and so on. Use whatever literal associations that appeal to you.

3. Do this for each of the seven chakras, and imagine breathing into each chakra.

If you have difficulty visualizing either the colors or the locations, try reclining and placing stones of the appropriate colors on the locations indicated on the diagram. Seeing the stones will help you hold the colors in your mind. The tactile sensation of the stones on your body will help you remember the locations. Stones can usually be found at either New Age shops or rock shops.

When you get comfortable with this visualization, and want to add intentions that relate to the function of each chakra, you can take this meditation as far as you choose. This is also a wonderful exercise to do with your parent, whether or not you identify it as a Chakra meditation. This can be used a way to help your parent relax, heal and move forward.

When you are complete with the visualization, take a few moments to feel your feet on the ground, wiggle your fingers, stretch, and return your awareness to the physical.

Enfolded by the Light

The above practices can be performed as either an extended meditation or a momentary shift to help you call back your awareness and remind yourself to take care of YOU. They need not take more than fifteen or twenty minutes. I find that when I am tired or stressed, it is often sufficient to simply stop, feel my feet on the ground, visualize myself enfolded in white light, instantly call-back or reclaim my energy, and continue. The whole affair takes less than a minute and helps me get through the moment, the hour, and finally the day.

It's easy to fall into the trap of believing that any time we take for ourselves during this process is selfish. But being self-ish is really nothing more than taking care of ourselves. In this context, it is not only healthy to pay attention to the "self," it is absolutely required. If we neglect ourselves, it always comes out in some other form: illness, resentfulness, feeling like a victim, snappishness, or subterranean anger than lurks and erupts at the most inopportune time and is disproportionately expressed.

Summary and Major Points

1. In addition to the usual ways we have of taking care of ourselves, methods that support our ability to manage our personal energy resources offer the strongest tools to keep us healthy, focused, and positive.

2. When we are concerned for others, multi-tasking, and running in different directions, our energy becomes scattered, leaving us with diminished resources.

3. Ways of maintaining physical and mental energy include:

- Proper nutrition: a diet filled with high quality protein and complex carbohydrates;

- Consuming least at eight glasses of water per day;

- Twenty-thirty minutes of daily aerobic exercise beyond the physical demands of packing boxes, etc.

4. In addition to physical and mental support, adult children moving their parents need to care for their own spirits. In caring for our parents it is all too easy to neglect our own spiritual needs.

5. Practices to care for the spirit include:

- Deep Relaxation or Meditation;

- Breathing and visualization to recharge the body's aura, or physical energy field;

- Energy re-claiming;

- Establishing healthy boundaries;

- Energizing and Clearing Your Power Centers (Chakras);

- Periodic grounding.

6. Self care is not the same as selfishness. Taking care of ourselves when moving our parents or in times of stress is essential to being able to handle the demands of the event.

7. Using these methods need not be time consuming. Any of the methods, once committed to memory, can be done in a heartbeat and incorporated seamlessly into daily activities.

Suggested Activities

1. Locate a water container that is convenient to take with you and to refill, as a way to help remind you to drink adequate water throughout the day.

2. Determine how you can build in some regular exercise into your routine.

3. Locate a quiet spot and try the Deep Relaxation technique. Each day, extend this practice until you are relaxing for fifteen to twenty minutes at a sitting.

4. Try the exercise for strengthening your energy field a few times in a quiet setting.

5. When you have memorized the technique, try a quick version of it whenever you need it and make a mental note of the results.

6. The next time you anticipate the need to establish some boundaries with your parents, visualize your energy balloon and set your intentions **before** meeting with them. Note the subtle differences in your interactions.

7. Practice a Chakra cleansing exercise for yourself to strengthen your own field to support you in your role as caretaker and helper. If your parents are open to this, talk them through the exercise. You don't have to mention Chakras, just use a color image to help them relax.

8. Try any one of these exercises whenever you have a moment, even if you just have time for the short version. The more you use them, the easier and most effective they become.

9. Share any of these you would like with your parents, using the language (religious, spiritual, or scientific) you feel will be most acceptable for them.

15 Moving Forward With Some New Thoughts

One of my favorite poems is "*Warning: When I Am An Old Woman*", by Jenny Joseph. I realize I am not alone in this and have thought about what it is that strikes such a chord in us. As you read it, see what it brings up for you.

> When I am an old woman I shall wear purple
> With a red hat which doesn't go, and doesn't suit me.
> And I shall spend my pension on brandy and summer gloves
> And satin sandals, and say we have no money for butter.
> I shall sit down on the pavement when I'm tired
> And gobble up samples in shops and press alarm bells
> And run my stick along the public railings
> And make up for the sobriety of my youth.
> I shall go out in my slippers in the rain
> And pick the flowers in other people's gardens
> And learn to spit.
>
> You can wear terrible shirts and grow more fat
> And eat three pounds of sausages at a go
> Or only bread and pickle for a week
> And hoard pens and pencils and beermats and things in boxes.
>
> But now we must have clothes that keep us dry
> And pay our rent and not swear in the street
> And set a good example for the children.
> We must have friends to dinner and read the papers.
>
> But maybe I ought to practice a little now?
> So people who know me are not too shocked and surprised
> When suddenly I am old, and start to wear purple.

Personally, I believe it's because the poem takes the eccentricities of old age and turns them into a badge of honor and—the little indiscretions we can look forward to. Having to be so responsible all the time can be a drag. As parents we became consumed with setting the right example, teaching our offspring how to be good citizens of the world, and upholding other myths about being the grown-ups. The result is that we often forget to have fun along the way. In the process, we also teach our progeny that this is what it's like to be the adult—no fun!

We got to be kids again in spurts when our little cherubs were in elementary school and we tagged along on field trips. But by the time they became pre-pubescent fifth graders, they didn't even want us showing up at school. Junior high brought, "Oh Mom, how *could* you?" Once they were in high school we were grinding our teeth at night, hoping they would get through driving, college applications, dating and sex without devastating consequences. Now our children have become adults (or nearly), and we can relax a little.

But wait, Mom and Dad are waiting in the wings and they now need us. The prize is always just around the corner—another step or two, and perhaps then we'll get to relax. No wonder we now fantasize about breaking the rules when we get older. Maybe then we will have both time and permission to ignore the rules (gobble up all the samples in stores), be frivolous (wear satin sandals), ignore convention (sit down on the pavement when we're tired) and do the outrageous (learn to spit). That time is now for our parents.

So, let us practice. In the midst of helping, let's break some rules. Let's go to the park with them, which is different from just taking *them* to the park. Let's have brownies for breakfast, take in a play, giggle when we feel like it. Let's find a way to enjoy our time with our folks, before it's too late for us and for them. And please, let's have fun with our kids, so they will know it's OK to be an adult *and* be fun and... hopefully, they won't get stodgy with us when WE get old.

We may need to modify some things along the way. Mom and I used to enjoy going to movies together, but now it's hard for her to understand the entire dialog because of her hearing loss. Some time ago I began to assume that meant movies were out, but she told me she still enjoys the event. We check out movies to watch at home, but these days I avoid the ones with accents, because I know she won't be able to follow those. We adjust.

When I turned sixty this year and my twenty-seven year old razzed me about getting old, he explained to my friends that if he and his brother stop joking with me, I'll get suspicious and actually believe that I've turned old. Perhaps it will happen so gradually, no one will notice that I wear funny shirts and satin sandals.

Out of the Mold

This past Christmas Mom and I found ourselves spending the day together without the rest of the family. One of my sons, Director of Ski Patrol at a resort on Mt. Hood, stayed on the mountain where the peak ski season had just started. The other was with his wife trying to do Christmas differently after the death of her own mother. Our Christmas day was quiet and non-traditional, a far cry from those we had each experienced in our younger days. Her retirement complex empties out during the holidays, so although she lives only thirty miles away, she spent the night with me on Christmas Eve. We enjoyed a movie, drank hot chocolate and had a sort of a slumber party. Christmas morning we slept late and drank good strong coffee as we put together a thousand-piece puzzle. It's something we both like to do and it allows time for conversation to emerge outside of those focused on necessities. It would have been easy to sink into the malaise that hits many of us on holidays that don't "measure up" to the hype. So we created something out of the mold.

Nothing But Time

For our parents, uninterrupted time with their grown children is possibly the greatest gift. Putting together puzzles isn't the full-tilt, hang-gliding variety of fun—but it's an enjoyable, non-structured sharing that invites spontaneous chat. Happy memories about my Dad burbled up, along with stories about granny chasing Mom around the cotton patch and me splitting my chin on the pogo-stick as a kid. These small intimacies were possible because we'd stopped the clock for a few hours. It's important.

We have a unique opportunity at this phase of life to look backward and forward at the same time. Yes, doors are closing. But others open. What piece of life have your parents not savored because they were busy being parents? How can we offer them another taste? What old memories or gaps in judgment might we heal simply by being emotionally present with them NOW, when they have the time to be there? Take time to smell the flowers—and yes, maybe even pick a few from the neighbor's yard.

One family I know, whose parents have just relocated nearby, has devoted a side yard to their parents' love of miniature trains. There are railroads and tunnels, ponds and whistle stops. It's a generous acknowledgement and allows them a way to continue with an activity that would not be possible in the retirement complex where they live. It also keeps the families in contact without there always having to be an event or planned visit.

I will never forget my mother's statement to me when I was getting all-efficient about how we would use our time on a particular outing. It was a statement of her life in the moment, "I have nothing *but* time."

A New Paradigm

We can teach old dogs new tricks. And I'm not talking about our parents. What we do here for and with our parents is the seed for creating a new model for ourselves. We are at a stage in history and in our lives when many paradigms are changing. The way we are aging is new. We *are* aging, but we are not becoming *old* at the same rate. My mother, quite aware of her 87 years and her infirmities, still says, "When I get old…" She is not yet old in spirit. She's a liberal, forward thinking, feisty woman, with a youthful spirit housed in an aging vessel.

The usefulness of the tools in this book extends far beyond the realm of helping our parents. Step by step, as I discovered each of them independently, applying them has changed the way I approach everything from parenting and career to my relationship with my family, friends and clients. When I divorced twelve years ago, I had no plan for my future; I was simply responding. I'd given up a career to say at home with my sons and had collapsed myself into the relationship. When I was introduced to Feng Shui and the model of the Nine Life Domains, I put it together with what I knew about the power of intention and applied the concepts to creating a vision of a new future. Adding Dispute Resolution I discovered a better model for handling the differences of opinion that are just a fact of life. The experience with Victim Services gave me compassionate ways to apply all of the other skills I'd learned. Piece by piece I began healing my life and learning how to do things differently. It took years to meld them into an integrated whole and to understand their transformative power regardless of age and stage of life. I hope they will bring you the same comfort and benefit.

I invite you to experiment with these tools beyond this event. The specific questions will vary, but each tool you've encountered in this book can stand alone and be called into play at any point during a project, encounter or relationship. One of the most exciting results for me has been to see my sons use them at an almost unconscious level to craft deliberate lives. Of course, they still face challenges, but they are sculpting their lives consciously, finding work that is intrinsically satisfying, and seeking soulful relationships.

When we are conscious enough to employ even *some* of these tools, *some* of the time, we dramatically shift the balance of life in a positive way. Collectively, the tools represent a system for living. Independently, they can act like the system of "checks and balances."

Looking Forward

Ushering my mother into the next stage of her life has plunged me into thinking about how we, as one of the largest single demographics in the world, can set into motion a different way of good-living during our twilight years, as our later chapters are often titled. Recently, the airline industry passed legislation extending the age of mandatory retirement for airline pilots from sixty to sixty-five. There are beginning to be nursing homes designed around what is called a residential model, as opposed to the previous standard known as the medical model. This is a step in the right direction.

I'd personally like to witness the creation of age-integrated communities where the elderly can live simply, cost effectively and productively, no longer segmented out to live only with "their own kind." Age segregation is boring and it's isolating. Further, young people need contact with older populations—to round out their view of the world, to provide continuity and to make us a more humane society. I'd like to see homes designed in such a way that we can age in place. Even the retirement communities I have seen built for that express purpose are incorporating only minimal adjustments like wheel chair access in the bathroom and grab rails in the tub and shower. We need more.

A Challenge

Daily, as I am with my mother, I try to slow down my internal clock. I want to remember our conversations and be aware of how her contributions have shaped my life. In knowing our parents more completely, we come to know ourselves and how we have become who we are. In acknowledging their struggles and easing those we can, we gather the knowledge and insights that help create a better future for ourselves and for our own children as they will face our aging just as we have faced that of our parents.

If we are conscious and compassionate collectively and recognize the gift in this difficult process, we hold the power to change *their* present and *our* future.

I leave you and your parents with a blessing for well being and a joyful, mutually enriching journey.

Epilogue

A couple of years ago, when Mom and I stumbled into the changing landscape of later life and began the tenuous discussion about her moving to a more manageable living space, neither of us knew where that journey would take us literally or figuratively. Although we anticipated a plethora of challenges, those that I'd somewhat planned for did not occur. Assuming Mom would live well into her 90s, I purchased a home with her in mind—one we could share when she could no longer live alone and might finally agree to move in with me. She had assured me, "It's not gonna happen," and she was right. We could not have predicted the road ahead or the blessings and challenges to be found along the way: the healing that took place in our own relationship, nor the surprising, new and dear friendships that emerged.

As I was writing the book, what was most profound for me was the way our relationship continued to evolve into one much richer that simply that of parent and child. Later developments brought with them even deeper insights and discoveries. My greatest hope for helping Mom was a genuine awareness of her physical and emotional needs and the ability to respond to those needs in a way that she could experience as caring. This required a mindfulness that made it necessary for me to step outside myself and to be exquisitely aware of every nuance so that I could also find ways to honor her spirit and emotions in the context of her needs. I wanted to be aware of and responsible for the dynamics I personally brought to the table and when necessary, change old patterns and find more helpful ones. This, essentially, became the basis for the book. There were a lot of dance steps to change, and pretty soon we learned to waltz—although sometimes awkwardly.

What I had not anticipated, but what occurred organically as a result of the process, was the healing of my mother's spirit. Mom, who for so long had denied herself the simple joys of allowing people to show how much they cared and of receiving acts of kindness without always having to reciprocate in bigger and better ways, finally allowed herself a bit of grace.

As Moving Your Aging Parents, went to print, life took a surprising turn. Mom was diagnosed with pancreatic cancer, a disease known for the speed at which it takes its immense toll. It is also known for something else in the community of alternative healers. A curious relationship between personality type and this cancer has been found and scientific or not, it seems the disease was found most often in people who have been unable to "taste the sweetness of life."

Medically speaking the pancreas is, in fact, an organ responsible for producing enzymes, pancreatic juices and the hormone insulin, which it then secretes into the blood stream in order to regulate the body's glucose or sugar level. Failure to metabolize sugar—the sweetness of life—was a perfect metaphor for the way Mom lived life. As we knew her, she had steadfastly refused the discussion of emotions, balked at the idea of "happiness," and had difficulty allowing others to do favors for her, even though she readily did favors for others. She was not one to ask for help (considered it a weakness) and was embarrassed when help was offered. She wrote a "thank you" note when she received a thank you note! And she preferred to visit someone in their home, because she could escape if the conversation turned personal or was laced with feelings she was unable or unwilling to confront.

Remembering back, I saw Mom soften as the process of her relocation and settling in to her new place progressed. When she realized my sister and I were not just going to "take over," she embraced this new partnering with her adult children, became more flexible, relaxed her judgments (a bit) and began to allow more friends and emotional intimacy into her world.

Once she was diagnosed and accepted it as real, she had a logical explanation for her encroaching frailty and began to see this as outside of her direct control. Somehow that made it more acceptable for her to receive help from others—though she persisted in writing a thank you note for every gesture of kindness. Her new friends embraced her—picked up books from the library, brought game day to her when she was felt like it, cooked meals, had stimulating conversations and read poetry. The help had always been available, but she had ever so politely declined, preferring to do without rather than expose her emotions. As time passed, she became able to recognize and accept it in the spirit in which it was offer: love. And it healed her, not physically, but it healed her spirit. For the first time in her life, I believe she was complete. For the first time, we could talk about how she had influenced our lives. Mind you, crying was still off limits, but we took liberties.

None of this might have occurred without the efforts she and we made to help her establish those relationships. Had she not made the effort to go to breakfast and game day, she would not have formed the bonds of friendship. Had she not been given and accepted the opportunity to share her wit and wisdom, her spirit and self-esteem would have withered and people would not have know her deep compassion, her bawdy sense of humor and human side. When newcomers came to the complex, she remembered her own sense of separateness and became the "greeter," showing them the ropes, teaching them the new games and encouraging them to connect. In the short time she was there, this diverse group of personalities—many of whom she had originally discounted because of their political or spiritual beliefs—became her friends and nurtured her in a way that she had not allowed in her previous life.

In all of the preceding years we had known her as our mother, we had recognized and come to accept her aloofness as part of her learned behavior and need to self-protect. But at the end, she met her death as the next adventure. I have had sufficient experiences with life-after-life that I know death to be but a transition. We were able to have open conversations about what she wanted, how the moment of passing might be and she was fearless.

She was complete and we—as a family were complete.

In "old days" it was common to hold a wake for the deceased person and everyone would tell their favorite tales and memories. In Mom's case, and at her request we held the "wake" to celebrate her life while she was still here to participate in the stories—and correct them! In her honor we mixed a batch of her favorite drink, Margaritas! All the family gathered and shared our favorite stories about times together and what her life had meant to each of us. And she seized the opportunity to correct us! Mom's Margarita Wake was a true celebration of her and I believe it contributed to her sense of completion.

The later years are rife with possibilities for stress and loss, but they are also an opportunity to make things right, to experience little joys in a way we might not have appreciated in our youth.

Take whatever time is available to you, whether it is a moment or a week or years to have the conversations about the real things. If the conversations don't come, simply listen with your heart. A door will open.

Appendix: Watch Lights

A Questionnaire to Help Decide When It's Time to Start Talking About Alternate Placement

Instructions: review each statement in Part I or Part II to evaluate your loved one's situation.

I. IF YOUR LOVED ONE CURRENTLY LIVES INDEPENDENTLY...

☐ Loved one has consistently lost weight and there is no medical cause for the loss.

☐ When you come for a visit, you find the stove burner on and unattended.

☐ Your loved one has made repeated errors in taking medication.

☐ EMS has been called to your loved one's home on more than once.

☐ Loved one is too confused to call for help.

☐ Increased frequency of illnesses or recent hospitalizations.

☐ Diagnosis of dehydration or malnutrition.

☐ Loved one refuses visits from family members in order to conceal deterioration.

☐ Individual's available funds are insufficient to cover sufficient private paid help.

☐ Medicine cabinet contains many bottles of expired medication.

☐ No longer able to cook nutritious meals for self.

☐ When asked to describe recent meals prepared, loved one relies heavily on cereals.

☐ Individual who is normally outgoing becomes socially withdrawn.

☐ Individual drives and doesn't know how they got somewhere.

☐ Neighbors report loved one wandering aimlessly around neighborhood or begging for food.

☐ You find thermostat set at extreme temperatures.

☐ Does not self-initiate a drink of water or meal preparation.

- [ ] Loved one has toileting accidents and is not able to care for self.
- [ ] Remains in pajamas most of the day.
- [ ] Deterioration in hygiene.
- [ ] Loved one neglects day-to-day business; stacks of unpaid bills inter-mingled with   advertising; clutter in home.
- [ ] Frequent complaints of lost personal items.

II. IF YOUR LOVED ONE CURRENTLY LIVES IN YOUR HOME...

- [ ] Loved one is too confused to call for help when left alone.
- [ ] Care needs for loved one are causing increasing conflicts with spouse and children.
- [ ] You find yourself consistently responding to loved one in an angry and impatient manner and later feel guilty for that anger.
- [ ] Care of your loved one is causing problems at your work place.
- [ ] You work and your loved one required 24 hour supervision.
- [ ] You come home to find your loved one has fallen or needed emergen-cy care and they were too confused to call for help.
- [ ] You are experiencing personal health problems due to the demands of care giving.
- [ ] You come home to repeatedly find the stove or coffee pot have been left on and unattended.
- [ ] Neighbors have found your loved one confused and wandering out-side.
- [ ] Deterioration in hygiene.

About the Author

Nancy Wesson is the owner of Focus On Space, a consulting firm serving clients in Austin, Texas and Washington, D.C. She is an International Speaker, Feng Shui Expert, Professional Organizer and Trainer who offers a toolbox of skills to achieve success through creating and maintaining mental, physical and spiritual spaces to support wellness, productivity, goal attainment and life-stage transitions.

Her interest in environments, health and the mind-body-spirit connection began after she received her Master's Degree in Audiology from the University of Texas. As an audiologist working with hearing-impaired clients, Nancy counseled patients regarding environmental adjustment to accommodate hearing loss and to improve quality of life. This experience prompted her to study the impact of environments on personal productivity, well-being and the management of personal resources.

Nancy's background as a Certified Mediator, Victim Services Counselor and Quantum Touch practitioner is integrated into every aspect of her work with both corporate clients and individuals. Her work with elders began in earnest during her tenure as Director of the Texas Medical Assistance Hearing Aid Program, which was mandated to deliver hearing aids and related services to qualified seniors.

Nancy has lectured on the topics of Environmental Factors in ADHD, Feng Shui, Organization, Aging and Elder Care, Time Management and Intuition at the University of Texas, U.S. Department of Labor, the U.S. Department of Justice, Shenandoah University, and the Texas Real Estate Commission as well as numerous seminars in both public and business venues. She has made guest appearances on KLRU public television in Austin, Texas and the Shenandoah University Television Production AT HOME. Her syndicated articles for the *Austin Homesteader* now appear on her website www.focusonspace.com

Nancy has authored and offers the following workshops:

- Creating Sustainable Environments for Elders;
- Environmental Adjustments for Special Needs;
- Environmental Factors in ADD/ADHD;

- Re-wiring the Brain
- The Whole Brain Approach to Managing Time, Energy and Personal Resources;
- Divorce Recovery;
- Feng Shui;
- Organizational Strategies;
- Re-wiring the Brain for Peak Performance;
- Arrange Your Listing for Success: Real Estate Feng Shui;
- Conflict Resolution for Non-Mediators;
- Balanced Living Through Design: Nine Steps to a Life You Love;
- Feng Shui and The Law of Attraction;
- Applied Intuition: Developing and Using Your Intuition.

Bibliography and Suggested Readings

Amen, D. (1998). *Change your brain, change your life.* New York: Three Rivers Press.

Barker, J. (1992). *Paradigms: The business of discovering the future.* New York: Harper Business.

Beck, M. (2003). *The joy diet.* New York: Random House.

Benson, H. (1975). *The relaxation response.* New York: Avon Books.

Brennan, B. (1987). *Hands of light.* Toronto: Bantam Books.

Breitman, P. & Hatch, C. (2000). *How to say no without feeling guilty.* New York: Broadway Books.

Bridges, L. (2004). *Face reading in Chinese medicine.* St. Louis: Churchill Livingston.

Campbell, D. (1997). *The Mozart effect: Tapping the power of music to heal the body, strengthen the mind and unlock the creative spirit.* New York: Avon Books.

Capacchione, L. (2001). *Power of your other hand: A course in channeling the inner wisdom of the right brain.* North Hollywood, CA: Newcastle Publishing Co., Inc.

Capacchione, L. (2000). *Visioning: Ten steps to designing the life of your dreams.* New York: Tracher/Putnam.

Choquette, S. (1994). *The psychic pathway,* New York: Three Rivers Press.

Day, L. (1996). *Practical Intuition.* New York: Broadway Books.

Dispenza, Joe (2007). *Evolve your brain: The science of changing your mind.* Deerfield, Florida: Health Communications, Inc.

Dickman, I. (1975). *No place like home: Alternative living arrangements for teenagers and adults with Cerebral Palsy.* New York: United Cerebral Palsy Association.

Dyer, W. (2004). *The power of intention.* Carlsbad, CA: Hay House, Inc.

Emoto, M. (2004). *The hidden messages in water.* Hillsboro, Oregon: Beyond Words Publishing.

Fisher, R. & Ury, W. (1981). *Getting to yes.* New York: Penguin Books.

Glassman, B. & Fields, R. (1997). *Instructions to the cook: A Zen master's lessons in living a life that matters.* New York: Bell Tower.

Green, B. (2003). *The elegant universe.* New York: Vintage Books.

Hannaford, C. (1995). *Smart moves: Why learning is not all in your head.* Arlington, VA: Great Ocean Publishers.

Jacobs, D. and Jacobs, R. (1999). *Zip your lips: A parent's guide to brief and effective communication.* New York: Houghton Mifflin.

Kingston, K. (1999). *Clearing your clutter with Feng Shui.* New York: Broadway Books.

Kohlberg, J. & Nadeau, K. (2002). *ADD-friendly ways to organize your life.* New York: Brunner-Routledge.

Leadbeater, C.W. (1985). *The Chakras.* Wheaton, Illinois: The Theosophisical Publishing House.

Lockwood, G. (1999). *The complete idiot's guide to organizing your life.* New York: Alpha Books.

Loehr J. & Schwartz, T. (2003). *The power of full engagement.* New York: Free Press.

McTaggart, L. (2002). *The field.* New York: Harper Collins.

Mace, N & Rabins, P. (2006). *The 36-hour day: A family guide to caring for people with Alzheimer disease, other dementias, and memory loss later in life.* Baltimore: The Johns Hopkins University Press.

Marcus, C. (1995). *House as a mirror of self.* Berkeley, CA: Conari Press.

May, E. (1966). *Independent living for the handicapped and the elderly.* Boston: Haughton Mifflin.

Monroe, R. (1977). *Journeys out of the body.* New York: Broadway Books.

Myss C. (1996). *Anatomy of the spirit.* New York: Three Rivers Press.

NAHB Research Center. (1996). *Residential remodeling and universal design.,* Washington, D.C.: U.S. Department of Housing and Urban Development, Office of Policy Development and Research.

Patterson, K., & Grenny, J. (2002). *Crucial conversations: Tools for talking when the stakes are high.* New York: McGraw Hill.

Patterson, K., Grenny, J., et. al. (2005*). Crucial confrontations: Tools for resolving broken promises, violated expectations and bad behavior.* New York: McGraw-Hill.

Pipher, M. (1999). *Another country: Navigating the emotional terrain of our elders.* New York: Riverhead Books.

Pink, D. (2005). *A whole new mind: Why right brainers will rule the future.* New York: Riverhead Books.

Robinson, M. (1993). *Be independent: A self-help guide for people with Parkinson's disease.* New York: The American Parkinson's Disease Association, Inc.

Rossbach, S. & Yun, L. (1994). *Living color: Master lin yuns guide to feng shui and the art of color.* New York: Kodansha International.

SantoPietro, N. (1966). *Feng Shui: Harmony by design.* New York: Perigee.

Shealy, C.N. (1999). *Sacred healing: The curing power of energy and spirituality.* Boston, MA: Element Books.

Sheldrake, R. (2003). *The sense of being stared at.* New York: Crown Publishers.

Sheldrake, R. (1999). *Dogs who know when their owners are coming home.* New York: Three Rivers Press.

Shulz, M.L. (1998). *Awakening intuition: using your mind-body network for insight and healing.* New York: Three River's Press.

Soyka, F. (1991). *The Ion effect: How air electricity rules your life and health.* New York: Bantam.

Thomas, K. and Kilman.R. (2002) Thomas-Kilman Conflict Mode Instrument, Mountainview, CA: CPP, Inc.

Vaughn, F. (1979). *Awakening intuition.* New York: Doubleday.

Wauters, A. (2002). *The book of chakras: Discover the hidden forces within you.* Hauppauge, New York: Barron's Educational Series, Inc.

Webb, M. (1997). *Dress your house for success.* New York: Three Rivers Press.

Wolfe, David, (2006) *Ageless marketing: changes in self perception across the life span.*
http://agelessmarketing.typepad.com/ageless_marketing/2006/08changes_in_self.html

Zander, R. & Zander, B. (2000). *The art of possibility.* New York: Penguin Books.

Index